So,
You're Going To
Try Marijuana

An Introductory Guide To

Buying And Using

Recreational and Medical Cannabis

(Without Being Embarrassed!)
2nd Ed.

By Ronan Blaschko

DISCLAIMERS AND LEGAL (CYA)
The Stuff You Acknowledge and Should Already Know.

This book is intended for informational and educational purposes only. The content provided does not constitute legal, medical, or professional advice. While every effort has been made to ensure accuracy, cannabis laws and regulations change frequently, and the author and publisher make no guarantees regarding the completeness or accuracy of the information provided.

The sale, possession, and use of cannabis and cannabis-derived products are regulated by law and vary across countries, states, and localities. It is the reader's responsibility to be aware of and comply with all applicable laws in their jurisdiction. The author and publisher do not endorse or encourage the illegal use, purchase, or distribution of cannabis products. Any discussion of cannabis-related products, including but not limited to Delta-9 THC, Delta-8 THC, CBD, and synthetic cannabinoids, is for informational purposes only and should not be interpreted as legal advice. If you have questions about the legality of cannabis in your area, consult a qualified attorney or official government sources.

This book does not provide medical advice. Cannabis products affect individuals differently and may carry health risks. The information in this book should not be used as a substitute for professional medical diagnosis, treatment, or advice. Before using any cannabis product, consult with a healthcare professional, especially if you have a medical condition, take prescription medications, are pregnant, or are nursing. The author and publisher assume no responsibility for any adverse effects resulting from the use or misuse of cannabis products.

Statements regarding cannabis, CBD, Delta-8 THC, and other cannabinoids have not been evaluated by the Food and Drug Administration (FDA). These products are not intended to diagnose, treat, cure, or prevent any disease. Individual results may vary.

Some cannabis products, including but not limited to Delta-9 THC, Delta-8 THC, and synthetic cannabinoids, are psychoactive and may impair cognition, coordination, and reaction times. Do not drive, operate heavy machinery, or engage in activities requiring full attention while under the influence of cannabis.

This book and its contents are intended for adult readers aged 21 and older (or the legal age for cannabis consumption in the reader's jurisdiction). The author and publisher do not encourage or condone the use of cannabis by minors.

This book does not provide financial, business, or investment advice. Any discussion of cannabis markets, business practices, or related industries is for informational purposes only. Readers should conduct their own research and seek advice from qualified professionals before making any financial or business decisions related to cannabis.

Not all cannabis products are created equal, and some may contain contaminants, unverified ingredients, or synthetic additives. Always purchase cannabis products from reputable sources and verify third-party lab testing for potency, purity, and safety. The author and publisher are not responsible for any negative experiences resulting from the use of unregulated or misrepresented cannabis products.

REVIEWS

"Man, I thought I knew my stuff, turns out I was a rookie. This book schooled me on things I didn't even know were options. If you think you've got cannabis all figured out, think again."
Don, West Coast Enthusiast

"I never smoked a day in my life, always thought it stank too much. But my doc said it could help me, and this book showed me ways to use it without ever lighting up. Now? Game changer."
Bobby, Southern Skeptic

"We were completely lost trying to figure out how to get medical cannabis for my mom. No clue where to start, what was legal, what wasn't. This book laid it out crystal clear. If you're in the same boat, this is your guide."
Tracy, Midwest Caregiver

"...First time I hit a dispensary, I was overwhelmed, so many choices, so little idea what to do. This book broke it down easy, so next time? I walked in like I owned the place and left with exactly what I needed."
Todd, East Coast Newbie

"It's like this book hijacked my brain, filled it with knowledge, and made me laugh while doing it. Now I know my way around a dispensary, and I smoke with confidence. Highly recommend."
Joey, Dispensary Regular

"I don't have time for boring books that ramble on. This one got straight to the point, gave me what I needed, and even made me laugh. Best recommendation I've gotten in a while."
Matthew, Impatient Reader

So, You're Going To Try Marijuana.

OTHER BOOKS AVAILABLE FOR THIS GUIDE

Also check out our extended version of the same information in our expanded Introductory Book described below. Each (**Guide or Book**) is available (or soon will be) in eBook, paperback, hardcover, and Audible formats.

(**This Guide**) **Condensed Version**: Labeled "<u>Introductory Guide</u>" with a man on the cover. This is a quick, no-nonsense (okay, maybe a little nonsense) Introductory Guide with bullet style, straight forward, concise facts and information for a reader who just wants the information without the long read.

Expanded Version: Labeled "<u>Introductory Book</u>" with a woman on the cover. This is the same information in an Introductory Book with expanded discussions on each topic in a conversational paragraph style format instead of bullets, targeted toward a reader who wants more of a paragraph book style read.

Both of these versions will walk you through everything you need to know about buying and using cannabis—whether you're looking for medical relief, a fun time, or just trying to avoid embarrassing yourself at a dispensary. Packed with actual facts, practical tips, and just the right amount of sarcasm, these guides will help you confidently navigate the legal market like a pro.

By the time you're done, you'll know what to buy, how to use it, and how to talk about it without sounding like someone who just Googled "what is weed?" So, if you're ready to achieve your marijuana goals without relying on questionable advice from your sketchy cousin's friend, this guide is for you.

OTHER SERIES

Also check out other "So, You're Going..." series from author Ronan Blaschko at www.RonanBlaschko.com.

ACKNOWLEDGMENTS

Published by Ronan Blaschko.
2965 28 ½ St.
Birchwood, WI 54817.
RonanBlaschko.com.

For inquiries, rights, or permissions, contact: Ronan@RonanBlaschko.com.

Printed in the United States of America. First Edition.

ISBN: 979-8-9927981-0-4.

To Those Who Made This Possible

Big shoutout to my college friends—or should I say fiends—for enlightening me on the "Highs" of life (pun fully intended). And an equally special thanks to my law career for dragging me through the "Lows" of what weed can do—because nothing kills a buzz faster than legalese and loopholes. But hey, thanks to this never-ending game of legislative whack-a-mole, even the non-smokers of the world now have a buffet of new, non-smoking ways to experience the magic of Mary Jane. Progress, right?

A heartfelt thanks to you, my dear readers, for not only buying this book (seriously, much appreciated) but also for being curious—and just bold enough—to dive headfirst into the weird and wonderful world of Cannabis. You've clearly heard the buzz (pun intended) and decided to see what all the fuss is about. That makes you my kind of people. Hopefully, this little adventure has introduced you to some new experiences, fresh perspectives, and, of course, a brand-new "Bud." Enjoy responsibly—whatever that means.

And finally—because no list of thanks would be complete without the most important person—I want to thank my incredible wife, Dana. Through every wild idea, ridiculous adventure, and probably more than a few moments that tested your patience, you've stuck by me. I couldn't do this without you, and honestly, I wouldn't want to. Your support, love, and ability to put up with my antics mean everything. You're my rock, my sanity (when I have any left), and the best adventure partner I could ever ask for.

Sincerely

Ronan Blaschko, Author

TABLE OF CONTENTS

Introduction:
Welcome to the Weed Renaissance

So, you're thinking about trying marijuana—or at least curious about its benefits—but the idea of diving into this wild, green world has you feeling a little hesitant. Naturally, you did the responsible thing: you bought a book to figure out how to get high—or, of course, to help your "grandmother" with her arthritis pain. Sure. We totally believe you. Wink, wink.

Well, congrats! You've either finally decided to embrace the wonders of cannabis, or—more likely—someone (a doctor, a cool nephew, or maybe a persuasive Reddit thread) convinced you that weed might help with your anxiety, pain, or crushing existential dread. And now, here you are, gripping this book like it holds the secrets to the universe. And honestly? It kind of does.

For decades, society has demonized cannabis, painting it as the gateway drug that would turn you into a jobless, couch-ridden snack monster with an insatiable craving for Taco Bell at 2 a.m. (Okay, that last part might be true, but is that really such a bad thing?) Then, at some point, lawmakers looked around, realized that weed wasn't turning people into deranged criminals, and—shocker— discovered they could make a boatload of tax revenue from it. And just like that, we entered what I like to call *The Great Weed Renaissance*.

So, Who Is This Book For?

If you've been puffing away since the days when a dime bag actually cost a dime, brace yourself—this ain't your grandma's homemade stash anymore. Today's cannabis is stronger, smarter, and will knock you on your ass if you're not careful. If you're still buying whatever your cousin's friend happens to have because "it's always worked," you're missing out on a world of strains designed to do more than just get you high—they can make you creative, relaxed, pain-free, or suddenly fascinated by the history of ceiling fans.

Maybe you're new to this and have no idea where to start. Maybe you smoked some mystery bag "oregano" back in college, had a paranoid meltdown, and swore off cannabis forever. Or perhaps you're here because your mom read an article about CBD curing everything from arthritis to a bad attitude and now wants you to be her personal drug dealer. Regardless of how you got here, this book is your nonjudgmental (and slightly sarcastic) guide to understanding, buying, and enjoying cannabis—without embarrassing yourself or accidentally calling 911 because you "forgot how to breathe."

Ever tried CBD that made you feel like a Zen master, only to buy another jar that did absolutely nothing? Welcome to the weird and wonderful inconsistencies of cannabis products. One batch can change your life, and the next has you questioning reality—mostly because you feel nothing. This book breaks down why that happens and how to stop throwing money at products that don't work.

Whether you're returning to cannabis after a long break, trying it for the first time, or just looking to stop blindly trusting Chad at the dispensary, this book will help you navigate the modern marijuana landscape with confidence (and fewer wasted paychecks).

What We'll Cover
(Besides the Obvious "How to Get High" Stuff).

What this book will do is help you understand what you're actually putting in your body, so you can get the experience you want instead of playing Russian roulette with your high. If you're ready to ditch the guesswork and upgrade your cannabis game, you're in the right place. This isn't just a "how to roll a joint" book (although, don't worry, we'll cover the many ways to enjoy marijuana products too). We're diving into the nitty-gritty details, like:

- What even is cannabis? (Besides something your weird uncle grows in his basement.)
- The difference between THC and CBD (and why one makes you giggle uncontrollably while the other just makes you feel mildly content with your life choices).
- The many ways to consume cannabis, from old-school smoking to fancy edibles that will have you questioning your entire existence.
- How not to overdo it and end up in a fetal position on your kitchen floor, convinced you've discovered the meaning of life but are too scared to move.
- Where to buy weed legally, so you don't end up making awkward small talk with a guy named "Trunk Tony" in a Walmart parking lot.
- What to do if you want to buy weed for your aging parents but aren't sure if you're legally allowed to turn Grandma into Snoop Dogg.

A Few Important Disclaimers:

Before we go any further, let's get a few things straight:

1. **I am not your lawyer.** No, I won't teach you how to smuggle edibles through airport security—figure that one out on your own. If you get arrested for trying to smuggle a pound

of weed in your carry-on, that's on you. (Also, why would you do that? This book literally has a whole section on how *not* to end up in jail.)

2. **I am not your doctor**. This is not a medical guide—if you're looking for a cure-all, call your doctor (or your neighborhood conspiracy theorist). Sure, we'll talk about how cannabis might help with pain, anxiety, and even sleep, but if you take medical advice from a book that also jokes about the joys of edible-induced existential crises, that's on you too.

3. **I am not your supplier**. This is also not an exhaustive list of every strain ever created or how to grow it, if that's what you want, just ask the dude at the dispensary who won't stop talking about terpenes.

4. **Cannabis affects everyone differently**. Just because your friend can smoke a whole joint and still function like a normal human doesn't mean you can. Start slow or prepare to have a very intense conversation with your houseplants.

Cannabis is fun. It's also complex, deeply misunderstood, and occasionally anxiety-inducing if you don't know what you're doing. But don't worry, you have this book, and I have just enough sarcasm and life experience to guide you through it.

By the time you finish reading, you'll know how to walk into a dispensary like a pro, find the right products for your needs, and *maybe* even convince your skeptical mom that weed is just fine (or at least not the devil's lettuce).

So, buckle up. You're about to take a journey into the world of cannabis—without the risk of getting lost in a dispensary for three hours trying to figure out what the hell a "terpene profile" is. Let's get started.

Chapter 1: Cannabis 101
A Crash Course Without the Crash

What Is Cannabis, and
Why Does It Have So Many Names?

Welcome to Cannabis 101, where we break down everything you need to know before you accidentally buy the wrong strain and end up on the couch the next morning with White Castle boxes all over the floor. This section will arm you with enough knowledge to confidently stroll into a dispensary, nod wisely at the budtender's recommendations, and pretend you've known what a "terpene profile" is your entire life.

If you've ever felt confused by the sheer number of words people use for cannabis—weed, pot, grass, ganja, the devil's lettuce (thanks, Grandma)—you're not alone. It's as if every generation decided to rebrand it just to mess with the next one.

For the record, cannabis is the correct term. It refers to the plant itself, which comes in a variety of forms, strengths, and legal headaches. Everything else—weed, pot, reefer, dank, Mary Jane—is just creative branding courtesy of stoners throughout history.

Now, let's get something straight: cannabis isn't one single thing. It's an umbrella term that includes different types of plants and chemical compounds, which leads us to...

Meet the Family:
Sativa, Indica, and Hybrid Explained

If you've ever stood in a dispensary staring at a giant menu labeled **Sativa, Indica, and Hybrid**, wondering if you should just blindly pick something and hope for the best—don't worry. This guide is here to prevent that disaster.

Sativa: The "Let's Get Stuff Done" Weed.

- Effects: Uplifting, energetic, creative.
- Best For: Daytime use, brainstorming, deep conversations about why we park in driveways and drive on parkways.
- Risks: May cause overthinking ("Why did I say that stupid thing in 2009?" syndrome).

Indica: The "Let's Melt Into This Couch" Weed.

- Effects: Relaxing, sedating, physically heavy.
- Best For: Nighttime use, unwinding, pretending you don't have responsibilities.
- Risks: You may wake up covered in Dorito dust wondering where the last four hours went.

Hybrid: The Middle Child of Weed.

- Effects: A mix of Sativa and Indica, depending on the strain.
- Best For: People who want SOME relaxation without turning into a human puddle.

- Risks: Strains vary wildly, so you might feel energized AND sleepy at the same time, which is... confusing.

Most dispensary menus now go beyond these categories and list **terpene profiles**, which is a fancy way of saying, "This weed smells nice and affects you in a certain way." But we'll get into that later. For now, just remember:

- Sativa = Get Up and Do Stuff.
- Indica = Sit Down and Forget About Stuff.
- Hybrid = Choose Your Own Adventure.

Pro Tip: A great way to remember the difference is Indica is "In Da Couch".

THC, CBD, CBN, CBG, CBC? High, Happy, Sleepy, Energy, Doc

So, what's the deal with these three-letter abbreviations everyone keeps throwing around? These are the dwarves of the Cannabis world. The best known are THC and CBD (which come from the same plant, but they do **very** different things. THC is psychoactive (translation: it messes with your brain in a fun way, the "High"), while CBD is non-psychoactive (translation: you can take it before a work meeting without accidentally launching into a 20-minute monologue about the nature of time, the "Happy").

If you've ever wandered into the world of cannabinoids, you've probably heard of CBD. It's the golden child of hemp, touted for its calming effects without the psychoactive baggage of THC. But what about its lesser-known cousins, CBN, CBG, and CBC? Are they worth your time, or just the obscure relatives at the cannabinoid family reunion? Let's break it down.

THC (Tetrahydrocannabinol): The Traditional "High".

The part of cannabis that gets you high, makes food taste amazing, and occasionally causes you to overanalyze the lyrics of every Pink Floyd song.

CBD (Cannabidiol): The Mainstream Star.

The chill cousin of THC. It won't get you high, but it might help you relax, ease pain, and tolerate annoying coworkers. CBD is the one everyone talks about. It's widely used for relaxation, pain relief, and inflammation reduction—without getting you high. Whether you're dropping it under your tongue, rubbing it into sore muscles, or infusing it into your morning latte, CBD has cemented itself as the go-to for those seeking cannabis benefits without the buzz.

> *Important*: *THC gets you high, CBD does not—but both can have powerful effects, so understanding what you're consuming is the first step to a smart cannabis experience.*

CBN (Cannabinol): The Sleepy Sidekick.

CBN is what happens when THC gets old—literally. As THC degrades, it converts into CBN, making it one of the most sedative cannabinoids around. It's often marketed as a natural sleep aid, helping users wind down without the grogginess of traditional sleeping pills. While research is still developing, early findings suggest that CBN may also help with pain relief and appetite stimulation. Just don't expect it to knock you out like a tranquilizer dart—it's more of a gentle nudge toward dreamland.

CBG (Cannabigerol): The Overachiever.

CBG is the "stem cell" of cannabinoids, meaning it's the precursor to both THC and CBD. Unlike CBN, which comes from THC's breakdown, CBG exists in young cannabis plants before transforming into other cannabinoids. It's gaining attention for its potential antibacterial, neuroprotective, and anti-inflammatory properties. Some users report that CBG provides a mild mood boost and focus enhancement, making it a promising option for daytime use—think of it as the espresso shot of cannabinoids.

CBC (Cannabichromene): The Underdog.

CBC is like that quiet genius in the corner who doesn't get much attention but is secretly solving all the world's problems. Instead of binding directly to CB1 receptors in the brain (which cause psychoactive effects), CBC interacts with other receptors, such as TRPV1 and TRPA1, which are linked to pain perception, inflammation, and mood regulation acting as a natural antidepressant which might make it one of the most underrated cannabinoids out there. It's also being studied for its potential role in neuroprotection and skin health. While it doesn't have the fame of THC or CBD, CBC is a team player in the entourage effect, enhancing the benefits of other cannabinoids.

CBL (Cannabicyclol): The Mystery Cannabinoid

CBL is like the awkward guest at the cannabinoid family reunion—nobody's entirely sure what they do, still, they showed up, so we'll include them. It's a non-psychoactive compound that's believed to form when THC is exposed to light or air for too long—basically, CBL is sun-damaged THC. Scientists are still figuring out what it's good for (besides confusing stoners), but early research hints at possible anti-inflammatory effects. Will it become the next CBD? Probably not. But one day someone will ask if your weed has CBL, and now you can nod like you know what they're talking about.

Beyond THC and CBD: hello THCV and friends

Now that we've covered the usual three-letter suspects, let's peek at the four-letter crowd. In cannabinoids like THCV (tetrahydrocannabivarin) and CBDV (cannabidivarin), that V is your hint for a varin homolog. Varins carry a three-carbon (propyl, C3) side chain instead of the standard five-carbon (pentyl, C5) tail you see in THC and CBD, and the plant builds them from divarinolic acid rather than olivetolic acid. Quick cue for your brain: no extra letter means pentyl (C5), V means varin/propyl (C3), and P—like in THCP—means heptyl (C7).

As for the mighty "P," yes, a seven-carbon side chain sounds dramatic, but in actual cannabis plants THCP shows up in trace amounts, i.e., not enough to move the needle for normal use. Translation for this guide: interesting chemistry, cool trivia, and safely outside the scope unless you're deliberately buying products labeled "THCP."

CBDV (Cannabidivarin):
The Brainy Cousin Doing Clinical Trials

CBDV is basically CBD's research-obsessed sibling—the one off at medical school while CBD is headlining wellness expos. It doesn't get you high, but scientists are paying serious attention to it for its potential in managing seizures, especially in epilepsy and autism-related conditions. You probably won't find it at your local dispensary, and it won't make you float into your couch, but it just might end up in a prescription bottle someday. Basically, it's the cannabinoid your neurologist would hang out with.

THCV (Tetrahydrocannabivarin): The Elusive Diet Weed

If THC and a protein shake had a baby, it would be THCV. Already known as the "diet weed," THCV is being studied for its potential to suppress appetite, boost energy, and help with blood sugar regulation. It's psychoactive, but not in the "why did I eat three burritos?" way—more like "let's clean the whole garage" energy. Found in rare African sativas and often in microscopic amounts, THCV is hard to find, pricey, and usually gone by the time you ask. On the plus side, it gives you something to hunt for besides your missing lighter.

CBGV, CBNV, CBCV: The Indie Rock Trio of Cannabinoids

Think of these as the secret B-sides of the cannabinoid catalog—unreleased tracks with weird names and cult followings. These "varin" versions of more familiar cannabinoids (CBG, CBN, CBC) are being explored for all kinds of possibilities, from anti-inflammatory effects to neurological benefits. You probably won't spot them on a product label anytime soon, but just knowing they exist gives you bonus points at your next dispensary trivia night. Are they life-changing? Maybe. Are they obscure enough to make you sound like an expert? Definitely.

Which One Should You Choose?

- Go with CBD if you want a reliable, well-researched option for relaxation, pain relief, and general wellness.
- Try CBN if you're struggling with sleep and need a nudge toward restfulness.
- Experiment with CBG if you're looking for a potential energy boost, focus enhancement, or gut health support.
- Don't sleep on CBC if you're looking for mood support, potential neuroprotection, or anti-inflammatory benefits.

How Do They Compare?

Cannabinoid	Known For	Best For	Psychoactive?
THC	Euphoria, altered perception, appetite stimulation	Fun, relaxation, creative exploration	Yes
CBD	Relaxation, pain relief, anti-inflammatory	Stress, anxiety, chronic pain	No
CBN	Sedative effects, sleep aid, mild pain relief	Insomnia, relaxation, mild pain	Slight (very weak)
CBG	Anti-inflammatory, antibacterial, focus boost	Energy, concentration, gut health	No
CBC	Mood regulation, pain relief, neuroprotection	Anxiety, depression, inflammation	No
CBL	Rare, degraded THC with unclear effects	Experimental curiosity, future research, feeling like a cannabinoid hipster	No
CBDV	Similar to CBD but potentially better for seizures and neuro issues	Epilepsy, autism spectrum disorders, "Wow, that's oddly specific" vibes	No
THCV	Appetite suppression, energy boost, possible blood sugar regulation	Weight loss, focus, biohacker bragging rights	Slightly (high doses)

For the adventurous, some products now combine CBD, CBN, CBG, and CBC to create a "full-spectrum" effect, allowing you to reap the benefits of multiple cannabinoids at once. As always, start slow, pay attention to how your body reacts, and enjoy the ride—without the paranoia.

Then there's **the entourage effect**, which sounds like a terrible reality show but is actually a real scientific concept. It means that THC, CBD and their lesser known cousins work better together than alone—kind of like peanut butter and jelly, but for your brain. The theory suggests that cannabinoids and terpenes amplify each other's effects, enhancing therapeutic benefits while potentially reducing unwanted side effects. So, if you're debating between isolated CBD and a full-spectrum product, consider this: would you rather have a solo musician or an entire orchestra playing for your endocannabinoid system?

THC: The Overrated MVP

Yes, THC is the psychoactive component in cannabis. It's what gets you high, makes you eat an entire pizza, and convinces you that your dog is definitely judging you. But here's where things get messy:

- The difference between, say, 18% THC and 30% THC isn't as dramatic as you think. Once you pass a certain threshold (around 15-20%), you're not necessarily getting "higher"—your body just processes it differently.
- Your tolerance, metabolism, and even what you ate that day affect how THC hits you.
- More THC doesn't mean a better high—it just means more THC. You wouldn't judge a fine whiskey purely on its alcohol content, would you? (If you would, please step away from the Everclear.)

However, if you've ever stood in a dispensary and picked your weed based on the THC percentage like you're shopping for the highest-proof vodka, congratulations—you've fallen for one of the greatest marketing scams in cannabis. Don't feel bad; we've all been there. You see those little numbers on the jar and think, higher number = better experience, like some kind of caveman logic applied to weed. But here's the truth: THC percentage isn't the god-tier measurement of how high you'll get.

Ever had a strain that's technically lower in THC but somehow hit way harder than that 30% powerhouse? The real magic? Terpenes. Think of them like the seasoning in a dish—sure, THC is the protein, but without terpenes, you're just chewing on a bland, overcooked steak. So next time you're at a dispensary, don't just chase the biggest number—ask about the terpene profile. Otherwise, you might as well be drinking gasoline and wondering why it doesn't taste like a fine bourbon.

Terpenes:
Because Weed Shouldn't Smell Like Just Skunk

Ah, terpenes—the unsung heroes of cannabis. Everyone's always yapping about THC and CBD like they're the only VIPs at this chemical party, but what about terpenes? Terpenes are the compounds that give cannabis its smell and taste, but they also shape your high in ways THC alone never could. You know how some strains make you giggly and social while others glue you to the couch, questioning whether that wall was always blue? That's terpenes at work.

These little aromatic compounds are the reason your weed smells like a pine forest, a citrus grove, or, occasionally, like your high school gym locker. But they're not just about smell—terpenes actually influence how cannabis affects you, which means choosing a strain based on THC alone is like picking a beer based purely on alcohol content. Sure, Everclear will get the job done, but do you really want to go down that road?

So, What the Hell Are Terpenes?

Terpenes are natural compounds found in plants, and cannabis is full of them. They're the reason oranges smell like oranges, lavender smells like relaxation, and pine trees smell like Christmas and bad camping trips. Cannabis produces terpenes in the same resin glands as cannabinoids (that's THC and CBD for those keeping score at home), and together they work to create each strain's unique effects and personality.

Some terpenes help you chill out, some wake you up, and some make your living room feel like an avant-garde art exhibit where your coffee table is suddenly fascinating. This phenomenon is called the entourage effect—a fancy way of saying that THC and CBD are a lot more fun when they bring their terpene friends along for the ride.

Why Should You Care?

Because terpenes can mean the difference between couch-locking yourself into oblivion or suddenly feeling inspired to clean your entire house at 3 a.m. If you've ever had an experience where the same amount of weed hits differently depending on the strain, congratulations! You've already met terpenes—you just didn't know their names.

Meet the Usual Suspects:
Common Terpenes and What They Do.

Just like your friends, some terpenes are chill, some are hyper, and some are just kinda there for the snacks. Here are the major players:

1. **Myrcene** (The Couch-Locker).

- Smells Like: Earthy, musky, and a little bit like cloves.
- Effects: Puts you in relaxation mode faster than a weighted blanket soaked in NyQuil.

- Found In: Mangoes, lemongrass, hops (so yes, beer and weed do have a common ancestor).
- Best For: People who enjoy naps, people who need naps, and anyone who's ever "accidentally" fallen asleep in the middle of a movie.

2. **Limonene** (The Mood Booster).

- Smells Like: Citrus—think lemon rinds, not the sadness of diet soda.
- Effects: Uplifting, stress-relieving, and sometimes it makes you believe you're actually going to start that project you've been putting off.
- Found In: Lemons, oranges, and the will to not let anxiety win.
- Best For: Monday mornings, existential dread, and days when your brain insists that everything is terrible.

3. **Pinene** (The Focus Enhancer).

- Smells Like: Pine trees, fresh air, and questionable camping decisions.
- Effects: Alertness, memory retention, and the ability to remember why you walked into the kitchen.
- Found In: Pine trees, rosemary, and your grandpa's aftershave.
- Best For: People who forget what they were talking about mid-sentence (so, most of us).

4. **Linalool** (The Chill Pill).

- Smells Like: Lavender, flowers, and that fancy candle your aunt won't stop talking about.
- Effects: Stress relief, relaxation, and possibly making you feel like a yoga instructor without having to do yoga.
- Found In: Lavender, mint, and bubble baths.

- Best For: Anxiety-ridden overthinkers, people who say "I need a vacation" at least once a day, and literally anyone who wants to relax without melting into the floor.

5. **Caryophyllene** (The Anti-Inflammatory Badass).

- Smells Like: Black pepper, cloves, and that little kick you get in spicy food.
- Effects: Pain relief, anti-inflammatory, and strangely good at handling stress.
- Found In: Black pepper, cinnamon, and BBQ sauce (no, really).
- Best For: People with chronic pain, people who insist that spicy food is a personality trait, and anyone who yells at their joints for existing.

6. **Humulene** (The Snack Blocker).

- Smells Like: Earthy, woody, and suspiciously like your favorite craft beer.
- Effects: Appetite suppression, anti-inflammatory, and making you question if you really want that third slice of pizza.
- Found In: Hops, sage, and (shockingly) cannabis—because of course, weed contains the one thing that fights the munchies.
- Best For: People who want the benefits of weed without raiding the fridge like a feral raccoon, anyone who's trying to cut back on stress eating, and that one friend who always insists they "just don't get hungry" (we see you, Linda).

7. **Terpinolene** (The Party Starter).

- Smells Like: A delightful mix of flowers, pine, and citrus—basically, like a spa that serves cocktails.
- Effects: Energizing, uplifting, and great for those moments when you suddenly must rearrange all the furniture at 2 a.m.
- Found In: Apples, lilacs, nutmeg, and the overwhelming urge to organize your spice rack.

- Best For: Creative types, social butterflies, and anyone who needs to turn their sluggish brain into a high-speed idea factory (just be prepared to get really excited about things that may not deserve it).

Terpene Profiles: Your Weed's Personality Test.

Every strain has a terpene profile, which is just a fancy way of saying "this is what's in here, and this is how it'll make you feel." It's kind of like a dating profile—some strains are exciting and energetic, some are calm and cuddly, and some just make you want to stare at the wall for three hours while contemplating the existence of life.

Strains With Similar THC Can Feel Completely Different:

Terpenes interact with THC and other cannabinoids to create different effects. The same 25% THC strain can either have you hyped up and creative or asleep by 7 PM—all depending on the terpenes.

- A 20% THC strain heavy in myrcene and caryophyllene will feel relaxing, body-heavy, and sedating.
- A 20% THC strain with limonene and pinene will feel energetic, social, and productive.
- Meanwhile, a 30% THC strain with low terpene content might just make you feel... high but kind of meh—like cheap vodka versus a finely crafted cocktail.

A typical terpene profile might look something like this:

- Myrcene – 0.8% (Relaxing, sedating).
- Limonene – 0.5% (Uplifting, stress-relieving).
- Caryophyllene – 0.4% (Pain relief, anti-inflammatory).
- Pinene – 0.2% (Focus, memory retention).

This means the strain is probably going to chill you out (myrcene) while also keeping your mood up (limonene) and helping with any aches and pains (caryophyllene). Basically, it's like getting a massage while also remembering where you left your keys.

The Pros & Cons of Caring About Terpenes.

✅ Pros of Terpenes:

- You can actually choose weed based on how you want to feel instead of just guessing and hoping for the best.
- They add flavor and aroma—because who doesn't want their joint to taste like a fruit smoothie instead of a burning twig?
- They might enhance medical benefits, like reducing anxiety, pain, or inflammation.
- They make you sound smart when you casually drop "Oh, I love this strain—its caryophyllene content is chef's kiss" in conversation.

✖ Cons of Terpenes:

- Some people are sensitive to certain terpenes, meaning instead of getting relaxed, you just get a headache, which is not the point.
- They degrade over time—which means if you leave your weed sitting out like a careless fool, you're gonna lose some of those nice aromas and effects.
- Finding the right combo can take trial and error, so expect to do some "scientific testing" (which, come on, isn't the worst problem to have).

The Smell Test:
Why terpenes matter more than high THC percentages.

THC percentage is like horsepower in a car—sure, it matters, but if the rest of the build sucks, it's just wasted potential. A well-balanced, terpene-rich strain at 18% can hit way harder and better than a dry, lifeless 30% THC strain that smells like lawn clippings.

So, next time you're shopping for weed, don't just go for the highest THC like a rookie. Find the right terpene mix for the high you actually want. Because if you're smoking just to flex a number, you might as well start measuring your beers by ABV and calling White Claw a "fine spirit."

Instead of obsessing over THC numbers, ask about the terpene profile. If the budtender stares at you blankly, congratulations, you've found a dispensary that treats cannabis like a gas station beer aisle—time to find a better one.

Terpenes matter. If you've ever wondered why one strain makes you feel like a creative genius while another turns you into a sentient couch cushion, terpenes are the answer. Whether you want to feel energized, relaxed, focused, or like a human marshmallow, understanding terpene profiles helps you get exactly what you need—without the nasty surprises.

Better indicators of a good high:

- Terpene percentages above 1-2% (higher is better)
- A strain's dominant terpenes (because limonene vs. myrcene = totally different vibes)
- A fresh, pungent smell (if it smells weak, the terpenes probably degraded, and you're smoking sadness)

And here's a pro tip: keep a journal. Track the profiles of the products you try and jot down the effects, so you can weed out the winners from the duds. That way, you're not just experimenting blindly—you're building your own personal roadmap to the perfect experience. Experiment with different terpenes and dosages, and soon enough, you'll be navigating the cannabis world like a seasoned pro!

So next time someone asks what strain you're smoking, don't just say "Uh, the green one." Flex a little. Say, "Oh, it's a high-limonene strain with a touch of pinene, great for creativity and focus." Even if you don't know what you're talking about, they probably won't either.

Full-Spectrum, Broad-Spectrum, and Isolate: The Three Amigos of CBD

So, you've decided to dip your toes into the CBD world but suddenly find yourself drowning in terms like full-spectrum, broad-spectrum, and isolate—like, seriously, why does this feel like studying for a chemistry test? Don't worry, I've got you. Let's break it down like you're picking out the right kind of tequila—because let's be honest, that's the level of decision-making we're working with here.

Full-Spectrum CBD: The Whole Party Pack.

Imagine full-spectrum CBD as a wild cannabis house party—everyone's invited, including CBD, THC (a little, but enough to cause some chaos), terpenes, and a whole mix of other cannabinoids. The idea here is that all these compounds work together in what's called the **entourage effect**, meaning they enhance each other's benefits like a perfectly balanced group of friends hyping you up on a night out.

✓ **Pros of Full Spectrum:**

- Strongest therapeutic effects due to all cannabinoids working together.
- Some say it's the most effective for pain, anxiety, and inflammation.
- Contains natural terpenes and flavonoids, which may enhance benefits.

✗ **Cons of Full Spectrum:**

- Contains THC (up to 0.3%), so yes, **you can absolutely fail a drug test.**
- The taste can be earthy—so if you hate the taste of plants, good luck.
- Legality varies depending on where you live (thanks, federal government).

Who's It For?

If you want the full experience and aren't worried about drug tests, full-spectrum is your go-to. Just don't be surprised when you pop positive on a test after *swearing* you "only took CBD."

Broad-Spectrum CBD:
Full-Spectrum's More Responsible Sibling.

Broad-spectrum CBD is like full-spectrum, but with THC kicked out of the party—it still has CBD, minor cannabinoids, and terpenes, but the THC has been carefully removed (or at least reduced to undetectable levels). Think of it like a "mocktail" version of cannabis: still flavorful, still fun, but without the potential regret of failing a drug test.

✅ Pros of Broad Spectrum:

- Offers some entourage effect benefits without THC.
- Won't get you high (unless you're high on life, of course).
- Less risk of failing a drug test (keyword: less, not zero—some tests are extra sensitive).

✗ Cons of Broad Spectrum:

- Not as effective as full-spectrum since THC plays a role in the entourage effect.
- Still might have trace amounts of THC, which could cause issues in very sensitive drug tests.
- Harder to find reliable, high-quality broad-spectrum products.

Who's It For?

If you want most of the benefits of full-spectrum but can't afford a surprise drug test result, broad-spectrum is the safe(ish) bet. It's like decaf coffee—close enough, but not quite the same.

CBD Isolate: The Control Freak of the Group.

CBD isolate is CBD, and only CBD. No THC, no other cannabinoids, no terpenes—just pure, unfiltered CBD, like a hermit who refuses to interact with anyone else. While it's great for people who want zero risk of THC in their system, it lacks the entourage effect, meaning it might not be as effective as full- or broad-spectrum.

✅ Pros of CBD Isolate:

- 99% pure CBD—nothing else to mess with your system.
- Best for people who get drug tested frequently (corporate warriors, I see you).
- No cannabis taste—great if you hate the earthy vibe of other CBD oils.

✗ Cons of CBD Isolate:

- No entourage effect, meaning it might not work as well.
- Processed more heavily, so some people prefer more natural options.
- Kind of boring (let's be real, it's the plain oatmeal of CBD choices).

Who's It For?

If you need CBD without any risk of THC contamination (*hi, government employees*), CBD isolate is your safest choice. Just don't expect it to hit quite like full- or broad-spectrum.

Will You Fail a Drug Test? Let's Be Real.

- Full-Spectrum? Yes. Even if it's just 0.3% THC, some drug tests are *hella sensitive.*
- Broad-Spectrum? Maybe. Most of the THC is removed, but trace amounts could trigger a positive test result. It's rare, but it happens.
- CBD Isolate? No. If you're getting pure CBD isolate, you're safe—just make sure your product is actually legit and not contaminated with THC (*because street-sourced brands exist*).

Choose Wisely, My Friend.

Picking between these three is like choosing between craft beer, light beer, and non-alcoholic beer—they all have a purpose, but the experience isn't quite the same. If you don't care about drug tests and want the strongest effects, go full-spectrum. If you want some benefits without the THC risk, broad-spectrum has your back. And if you just need CBD and nothing else, isolate is the way to go—just know you're missing out on the full experience.

At the end of the day, know your body, know your job's drug policy, and for the love of all things green, buy from a reputable brand.

Understanding THCA: The "Non-Psychoactive" Twin of THC

Ever walked into a dispensary and seen something labeled "THCA" and thought, "Wow, they're just making up new letters now"? You're not alone. If you've been shopping for cannabis products, you may have noticed THCA (or sometimes THC-A or THCa) popping up everywhere. It sounds a lot like THC, so what's the deal? Are they the same thing? Not quite. THCA (tetrahydrocannabinolic acid) is like the Sneaky Cousin of THC That's (Sort of) Legal—until you apply heat, at which point it drops the act and turns into the mind-altering troublemaker we all know and love.

THC vs. THCA: What's the Difference?

When cannabis is fresh and unheated, it primarily contains THCA (tetrahydrocannabinolic acid) which is the raw, non-psychoactive precursor to THC (tetrahydrocannabinol).

Think of THCA as THC in its natural, raw form. When cannabis is freshly harvested, it's loaded with THCA, not THC. This means if you were to nibble on a raw nug (not recommended—very leafy), you wouldn't get high. That's because THCA has this little molecular tag—scientists call it a **carboxyl group** (science talk for a little molecular add-on) that prevents it from binding to your brain's cannabinoid receptors, but let's just call it a "buzz blocker."

However, the biggest difference between THC and THCA comes down to one thing: **heat**. Once you light it, vape it, or cook it, that buzz blocker burns away in a process called **decarboxylation** (a fancy word for "heat turns it into real THC"), and BAM—you're officially high. So, in other words, THCA is basically THC with a built-in delay button that activates the second you apply heat.

Effects: Will THCA Get You High?

Short answer: Not unless you heat it. Raw THCA won't deliver the euphoric, mind-altering effects that THC does. However, it is being studied for its potential therapeutic benefits, such as anti-inflammatory and neuroprotective properties. Some people juice raw cannabis leaves for THCA, hoping to gain medicinal benefits without the high. But if you plan to smoke, vape, or cook with it, THCA is essentially just THC waiting to happen.

Legal Loopholes: The THCA Gray Area.

Now, here's where things get interesting. Because THCA isn't technically psychoactive in its raw form, it has somehow sneaked past certain legal restrictions—at least for now. Some states allow high-THCA products because, on paper, they're *not* THC. But the second you apply heat and turn that THCA into actual THC, the legal landscape changes faster than a politician's campaign promises.

Federal law says hemp products are legal if they contain less than 0.3% THC—but that doesn't always factor in THCA's sneaky transformation abilities. This has led to dispensaries selling high-THCA flower under the guise of legality, knowing full well their customers aren't buying it to sprinkle raw on a salad. THCA's status is more of a loophole than a fully recognized exemption.

Buying & Using THCA
Without Accidentally Committing a Crime.

- **If you want to get high:** Go for THCA flower or concentrates—just know *that ONCE HEATED, IT'S LEGALLY THE SAME AS THC.*
- **If you want "medicinal benefits" without the high:** Stick to THCA tinctures, capsules, or raw cannabis juice. Though, let's be real—most people aren't juicing weed unless they have a wellness blog.
- **If you want to stay legal:** Research your state laws carefully, as some places are cracking down on THCA sales now that they realize their conversion potential. Just because a store sells it doesn't mean your local law enforcement understands the loophole—or cares.

THCA Is Basically THC in Disguise:
Know Before You Light Up.

THCA is like a kid wearing a fake mustache trying to get into an R-rated movie—it might fool the ticket guy for now, but once the lights come on, everyone knows what's up. If you're looking for a legal workaround, THCA might work—just don't be surprised if lawmakers crack down once they realize they accidentally legalized it. Until then, enjoy your *totally legal* THCA... just, you know, maybe don't announce it to the cops.

The Acid B-Squad: CBDa, CBGa, and Friends

- THCa isn't the only one sneaking around with a little "a" at the end. Meet its acidic cousins—CBDa, CBGa, CBCa, and THCVa. These are the raw, unheated forms of their better-known counterparts.
- They won't get you high either (sorry), but they're showing promise in the world of non-psychoactive wellness. Scientists are still figuring out what they do—so far we've got hints of anti-inflammatory, anti-nausea, and general good-vibes-without-the-buzz potential.
- Think of them as cannabinoids that haven't finished puberty yet. They're still useful, just not fully grown into their final form.

   Warning: If someone hands you a strain labeled "Couchlock," don't plan on being productive for the next few hours (or, who are we kidding, the rest of the day).

Delta-9, Delta-8, and the Other Deltas: What's the Difference?

If you've ever walked into a dispensary (or scrolled through the wilder corners of the internet), you've probably seen products labeled Delta-9, Delta-8, maybe even Delta-10 or something else that sounds like a secret military project. But what do these numbers actually mean? Are they all just different versions of THC? And—more importantly—are they legal where you live? Let's break it all down.

Delta-9 THC:
The Classic, The Legend, The One You Know.

Delta-9 tetrahydrocannabinol (THC) is the OG psychoactive compound in cannabis—the one responsible for getting you high. It's what you're dealing with when you buy traditional marijuana in a dispensary. Delta-9 interacts with your CB1 receptors, producing euphoria, relaxation, hunger (hello, munchies), and sometimes a little paranoia if you overdo it.

Delta-9 occurs naturally in cannabis, and its legality depends on your state. In some places, it's fully legal for recreational use. In others, only medical patients can buy it. And in some states, it's still totally illegal—though that hasn't stopped some creative workarounds (cue Delta-8).

Delta-8 THC: The Legal Loophole (Sort Of).

Ah, Delta-8—THC's laid-back cousin who shows up to the party in flip-flops and somehow never spills his drink. It's psychoactive, sure, but it doesn't hit you like a freight train the way Delta-9 can. Instead, people say it's more of a smooth ride—relaxing, a little euphoric, and with significantly less of the "Oh no, did I forget how to breathe?" moments that traditional THC can sometimes bring.

But here's where things get fun: Delta-8 is naturally found in cannabis, but in such tiny amounts that trying to extract it directly would be like trying to fill a bathtub with morning dew. So, what do manufacturers do? Science the hell out of it. They take CBD from hemp (because that's totally legal under the 2018 Farm Bill) and transform it into Delta-8 through a chemical process that sounds complicated but basically boils down to mad scientist meets legal loophole.

So, can you buy Delta-8 in states where Delta-9 THC is illegal? Surprisingly, yes—at least in a lot of states. Thanks to a legal loophole big enough to drive a dispensary truck through, Delta-8 exists in a weird gray area where it's technically legal even in places that clutch their pearls at traditional THC. But don't get too excited—some states have wised up and decided to slam the door shut, banning Delta-8 right alongside its notorious cousin. Basically, if lawmakers think Delta-9 is the devil's lettuce, they're not too thrilled about its slightly milder, legally ambiguous sibling either.

And that, my friends, is why Delta-8 exists in a delightful legal gray area. Since it's technically hemp-derived, producers argue it's fair game. Federal regulators, on the other hand, are still trying to decide if they should crack down or just let people enjoy their mildly buzzed, anxiety-free afternoon. Stay tuned.

Synthetic THC:
Delta-10, HHC, and Other Cannabinoid Spin-Offs.

As laws shift, new compounds pop up, offering fresh ways for both seasoned stoners and canna-curious newcomers to experience the plant. Most of these are made by modifying hemp-derived CBD, so they fall into the same legal gray area as Delta-8—for now.

Now, let's talk about lab-made THC—the truly synthetic stuff that doesn't naturally occur in cannabis at all. This includes compounds like K2, Spice, and other synthetic cannabinoids that have been linked to some seriously bad reactions (we're talking seizures, hallucinations, and ER visits). Because the cannabis industry loves a loophole, other THC variants have popped up, including:

- Delta-10 THC – Like Delta-8, but even milder. Often described as "more energizing."
- HHC (Hexahydrocannabinol) – A hydrogenated form of THC that's allegedly stronger and longer-lasting.
- THC-O – A synthetic cannabinoid that's reported to be 3x stronger than Delta-9 THC (and a little mysterious).
- THCP – A newly discovered cannabinoid, typically synthetically derived from hemp, with up to 33 times stronger binding to CB1 receptors than THC.

These cannabinoids initially slipped through the 2018 Farm Bill's loophole by being derived from hemp—until regulators caught on and started cracking down.

THC-O and THCP are among the most potent of the bunch, with THC-O often called the "psychedelic cannabinoid" for its intense, almost hallucinogenic effects, while THCP's ultra-high CB1 binding suggests it could be significantly stronger than regular THC.

Unlike Delta-8, which is naturally derived from hemp, fully synthetic cannabinoids—lab-made compounds designed to mimic THC—interact with receptors far more aggressively and unpredictably. You don't want this. Ever.

- Stick to regulated dispensaries—if you're buying from a gas station or bargain-bin bud portal website, be suspicious.
- Look for lab testing—legit brands will show third-party lab results verifying cannabinoid content.
- Avoid anything labeled as a "legal high" without proper ingredients listed.

Tips for Buying Delta Products
(And Not Getting Scammed).

- Check the legality in your state – Laws are shifting fast, and some states have banned Delta-8 even if they allow CBD.
- Buy from reputable sources – Stick with dispensaries and brands that provide lab-tested products.
- Be cautious with potency – Delta-8 is milder than Delta-9, but it can still get you high—so don't assume you need to double the dose.
- Watch out for synthetic junk – If it's labeled as "legal weed" and comes in an unverified vape or edible from a gas station, it might not be actual cannabis.

After All That, What Should You Try?

- If you live in a legal state, stick with traditional Delta-9 THC from a dispensary. It's the most natural and well-studied.
- If THC is illegal in your state, Delta-8 might be a legal option—but check your local laws first.
- If you want a milder high, Delta-8 is worth a try.
- Avoid trap-level synthetic THC—if you see something called "Spice" or "K2," run the other way.

As always, start low, go slow, and know what you're consuming—because not all THC is created equal.

> *Pro Tip*: keep a journal. Track the profiles of the products you try and jot down the effects, so you can weed out the winners from the duds.

Hemp:
The Unsung Hero of the Cannabis World

If cannabis were a family, hemp would be the responsible older sibling who holds down a steady job while THC is out partying. It's been around for thousands of years, used for everything from rope to clothing to food. But when it comes to buying and using cannabis, do you actually need to know about hemp? Absolutely. Here's why.

What Is Hemp?

Hemp is a variety of the Cannabis sativa plant that naturally contains very low levels of THC—less than 0.3% by law in the U.S. This means you can't get high from smoking hemp (unless disappointment counts as a psychoactive effect). However, hemp is incredibly versatile and a major player in the cannabis industry because it can be used to create:

- CBD products (oils, gummies, topicals, etc).
- Delta-8 THC (through chemical conversion of hemp-derived CBD).
- Textiles, paper, bioplastics, and even car parts.

Essentially, if cannabis has a "mainstream" side, it's hemp.

How Does Hemp Relate to Cannabis and THC?

Hemp and marijuana are genetically the same plant, but their key difference is THC content:

- Marijuana is cannabis grown for its THC, the compound that gets you high.
- Hemp is cannabis grown with almost no THC, often cultivated for fiber, seeds, and CBD.

Here's where hemp pulls a sneaky move into the world of recreational cannabis. See, most CBD products come from hemp—not because it's better, but because it's legal to grow and extract cannabinoids from it without the DEA throwing a fit. But the real plot twist? Those trendy Delta-8 THC, Delta-10, and HHC products that claim to get you high without technically breaking the law?

Yeah, they're usually made by chemically tweaking hemp-derived CBD into something that acts like THC but can still squeeze through legal loopholes in states that frown upon the real stuff. So even if you're a hardcore THC purist, there's a good chance hemp is lurking somewhere in the background, playing an unexpected role in your buzz.

Do You Need to Care About Hemp When Buying Cannabis?

Yes—depending on what you're buying.

If You're Buying CBD:

- You're almost always getting hemp-derived CBD, which is federally legal and widely available.
- Hemp-derived CBD is the same as marijuana-derived CBD, just with no THC.

If You're Buying Delta-8 or Other "Alternative" THC Products:

- These products likely came from hemp-derived CBD first and were chemically converted.
- Quality can vary, and some products may contain residual solvents or impurities—so always check lab tests.

If You're Buying THC in a Legal State:

- Hemp isn't a factor here—your Delta-9 THC is coming straight from marijuana.

- However, if you see "hemp-derived Delta-9 THC" (yes, it exists), it's a product that contains just enough THC from hemp to stay within legal limits but still produce mild effects.

Your Bar Sells THC? Yep, It's the Hemp Loophole

Ever wonder how you're sipping a 10mg THC seltzer in a bar in a state where weed is totally illegal? Surprise: it's because that THC was squeezed out of hemp.

Thanks to federal law, hemp-derived THC is treated differently—even if it gets you just as baked. So yeah, that "hemp beverage" in your fridge isn't fooling anyone. It's basically pot in a business suit.

This legal magic trick is why you'll find THC drinks, gummies, and vapes on store shelves across the country—even in states that still think "reefer madness" was a documentary.

So, Is Hemp Just a Loophole or Actually Useful?

Hemp is both a legal workaround and a valuable plant in its own right. It's responsible for bringing CBD, Delta-8, and other cannabis compounds to markets that otherwise wouldn't have access to them.

If you're buying THC products, it's important to know where they come from—hemp-derived THC may be legal in your state, but it's not the same as traditional cannabis-derived THC. And if you're looking for a non-intoxicating option, hemp-derived CBD is a solid choice.

In short, hemp is the boring but incredibly useful side of cannabis—like the straight-A student in a family full of wild siblings. And whether you realize it or not, it's probably already part of your cannabis experience.

Finding THCV: "The Diet Weed"
The Skinny Stoner's Secret Weapon

Alright, let's talk about THCV (tetrahydrocannabivarin)—because the cannabis industry loves long, complicated words that sound like something out of a mad scientist's lab. You may have heard about THCV, often called "diet weed," which is a tragedy for those of us who consider snacking an essential part of the high experience. Unlike THC, which turns you into a human vacuum for pizza rolls and peanut butter straight from the jar, THCV is more likely to make you forget that food exists.

THCV is like THC's skinnier, more energetic cousin who doesn't stick around for long. If THC is the laid-back dude on the couch, THCV is the one bouncing around the room asking if anyone wants to go for a jog. It's found in trace amounts in certain sativa strains, especially those from Africa (because apparently, the cannabis gods decided Americans didn't need this miracle molecule). Unlike THC, which binds directly to your CB1 receptors to get you high, THCV actually blocks those same receptors at low doses, which means it won't get you high unless you consume a lot.

So, why should you care about THCV? Well, here's what it supposedly does:

- **Suppresses appetite**. Great if you're on a diet, terrible if you enjoy stuffing your face while binge-watching nature documentaries.
- **Provides energy and focus**. Some users say it's like cannabis mixed with an espresso shot (but without the impending anxiety attack).
- **May help with diabetes and insulin resistance**. If the FDA ever decides to care about cannabinoids, this might actually be a big deal.
- **Acts as a neuroprotectant**. Science suggests it could help with conditions like Parkinson's disease, but let's be real—most people want to know if it'll make them giggle or pass out.

- **Doesn't last long**. The high from THCV is usually short-lived, so don't expect to be flying for hours like you would with a heavy indica.

THCV promises energy, focus, and—brace yourself—zero munchies. Yes, a cannabinoid that supposedly stops you from inhaling an entire pizza post-smoke. Realistically—THCV sounds too good to be true. A cannabis compound that doesn't make you eat everything in sight, keeps you alert, and might even help regulate blood sugar? Come on, that's basically sorcery. But before you sprint to the dispensary in excitement, let's talk about why THCV keeps mysteriously disappearing from shelves faster than your willpower around a bag of chips.

THCV isn't as easy to find as THC or CBD.

So, you've heard about this magical diet weed, and now you want to buy some? Well, good luck. THCV has been vanishing from dispensary shelves faster than a free sample tray at a weed convention. If you walk into a dispensary and ask for THCV, you might get a blank stare or a half-hearted attempt to upsell you on something else.

If you've noticed that dispensaries once stocked THCV and then quietly stopped carrying it, congratulations—you're paying attention. Minnesota, for example, sent sternly worded letters to almost 4,000 cannabis retailers in 2024, essentially saying, "Hey, stop selling that." (Because nothing makes people want something more than telling them they can't have it.) Over in California, regulators cracked down on hemp-derived cannabinoids, lumping THCV in with other forms of THC, because why let people have nice things?

Here's where things get tricky. While THCV along with lesser known cannabinoids CBDV, CBGV, CBNV and CBCV (being studied for medical benefits) are technically legal under the 2018 Farm Bill (as long as it comes from hemp with less than 0.3% THC), states get to make their own rules. Some states are totally cool with it, while others are treating THCV like it's plotting world domination. Your best bet?

- Check Your Local Laws – Because nothing kills a buzz like realizing you just bought an illegal product.
- Ask Dispensaries – If they have it, great. If they don't, enjoy the confused look from the budtender.
- Online Retailers – Some hemp-derived THCV products are sold online, but be prepared to decode vague marketing language like "high-energy cannabinoid blend." Just be sure you're not accidentally buying snake oil.

THCV: The Elusive Unicorn of Cannabis
Rare, Mysterious, and Worth the Hunt

THCV is a fascinating cannabinoid that's slowly making its way into the mainstream, but it's still a bit of a unicorn in the dispensary world. If you find flower with actual THCV levels worth mentioning, congratulations—you've hit the jackpot. It's rare, but some strains naturally produce it in slightly higher quantities. If you manage to find it, expect to pay a premium for the privilege of not getting the munchies. On the flip side, if you ever wanted a weed that might help you stay fit, THCV just might be your best friend. Or your worst enemy, depending on how much you love pizza.

Look, if you want a high that makes you feel like drinking green juice instead of devouring a cheeseburger, THCV is worth tracking down. If you prefer your weed to come with snacks and naps, maybe just stick with regular THC. Either way, THCV is an exciting cannabinoid—if you can find it before it vanishes again.

Moral of the story? THCV is like that mysterious friend who only shows up when they feel like it—hard to get, exciting when you do, and possibly life-changing. Or at least diet-changing.

The Science of the High:
How Weed Works in Your Body

Time for a little science lesson—but don't worry, I'll keep it short and fun so you don't feel like you accidentally wandered into a college lecture.

Your body has something called **the endocannabinoid system (ECS)**, which is basically a network of receptors specifically designed to interact with cannabis. Yes, you read that right—your body was literally built to process weed. If that's not proof that nature wants you to enjoy yourself, I don't know what is.

So, let's talk about your Endocannabinoid System—or as I like to call it, the secret control panel of your body that nobody told you about in health class. The ECS is basically your body's master regulatory system, responsible for keeping everything in balance, aka homeostasis (big word, simple meaning: keeping you from falling apart). It's like the thermostat in your house, making sure you're not too hot, not too cold, but just right—except instead of temperature, it helps regulate mood, sleep, pain, appetite, immune function, and whether or not you'll stress over that email you sent two days ago.

Your body actually makes its own cannabis-like compounds—yes, you naturally produce cannabinoids. Wild, right? These are called endocannabinoids (because they come from inside you, not a plant). They float around, binding to special receptors (CB1 and CB2) that are scattered all over your brain, immune system, and basically everywhere else. Think of them like tiny messengers delivering balance updates to your body. If something is off—like stress, inflammation, or your inability to handle slow walkers at the grocery store—your ECS jumps in to bring things back to normal.

Now, when you use cannabis, the THC and CBD hijack this system in the best way possible. THC fits into the CB1 receptors like a key in a lock, which is why you suddenly feel euphoric, relaxed, or, you know the vibe, deeply invested in the meaning of your pet's facial expressions. When you use cannabis, THC binds to receptors in your brain, causing effects like:

- **Euphoria** (Wow, I suddenly love everything.)
- **Relaxation** (I could stay in this chair forever.)
- **Hunger** (Everything in the fridge must be eaten immediately.)
- **Deep thoughts** (What if our entire universe is just one big simulation?)

CBD, on the other hand, doesn't bind to the same receptors. Instead, it works behind the scenes, reducing inflammation, stress, and overall crankiness. This is why CBD is legal pretty much everywhere (including places where THC is still banned by people who clearly need to smoke some).

CBD is more of a background operator. It helps regulate everything, kind of like the chill friend who diffuses drama at a party. Together, they work with your ECS to help with pain, anxiety, sleep, and making movie nights way more interesting.

So, next time someone tells you that cannabis is unnatural, remind them that your body literally has a system designed to work with it. Science, my friend—it's on your side.

How Different Strains Affect You
(Avoiding a Weed-Induced Identity Crisis).

If you've ever heard someone say, "This strain will make you feel RELAXED BUT FOCUSED," and thought, HOW IS THAT EVEN POSSIBLE? Welcome to the wild world of cannabis strains.

Strains are like wine: some are light and energizing (think Sauvignon Blanc), some are rich and heavy (think Cabernet), and some will straight-up knock you on your ass (think Everclear).

Each strain has different levels of THC, CBD, and other compounds called terpenes, which affect everything from taste to effects. We already went through the 7 popular terpenes earlier in this chapter.

To find the right strain, ask yourself:

- Do I want to be energized or relaxed?
- Do I want a strong high or just a mild buzz?
- Do I need to function, or is it okay if I spend the next three hours giggling at my own reflection?

Most dispensaries label strains based on these effects, but ALWAYS ask the budtender for guidance. Otherwise, you might accidentally take a "relaxing" strain at 10 a.m. and end up napping through an important meeting.

What we learned:
You Now Know Just Enough to Sound Smart

Alright, champ, before you go blazing into the great unknown, let's have a little chat about mindset. This isn't just some casual snack—you're about to alter your perception of reality (hopefully in a fun way). If your brain is running on anxiety, paranoia, or some deep-seated fear that your third-grade teacher is still disappointed in you, marijuana is going to amplify that.

By now, you should have a basic understanding of cannabis, THC vs. CBD, different strains, and why your body was apparently designed to enjoy weed. So, before you inhale deeply and start questioning your own existence, set your intention. Are you here to chill? Laugh at cat videos? Stare at the fridge for an hour? Good. But if you're secretly harboring unresolved drama, maybe save the weed for another day.

In the next section, we dive into everyone's favorite buzzkill— the law. Yep, before you start living your best cannabis-infused life, you might want to know how to buy legally and, more importantly, how to stay out of jail. Because we can all agree, orange jumpsuits are not a vibe. So, stay tuned, pay attention, and maybe take notes—because "I didn't know" doesn't hold up well in court.

> *Pro Tip*: Sativa = "Let's clean the whole house at 2 a.m." Indica = "Let's melt into this couch and contemplate existence." Hybrid = "Let's see what happens."

Chapter 2:
The Law, the Loopholes, and How Not to Get Arrested

Ah, the legal side of cannabis—a delightful maze of contradictions, loopholes, and "wait, that's illegal?" moments. You'd think that in a country where you can legally buy alcohol (which kills people) and cigarettes (which also kill people), cannabis would be a no-brainer. But no. Instead, we have a patchwork of confusing state laws, federal paranoia, and a whole bunch of ways to accidentally commit a crime just by existing near a dispensary.

So, let's break it down: what's legal, what's not, what's *technically* legal but still bootleg as hell, and how to avoid starring in your own episode of *Cops*.

> *Important*: *Congratulations! You live in an era where weed is legal in many places, taxed like crazy, and no longer something you have to buy from a guy named "Sketchy Steve" behind a gas station.*

Where You Can (and Can't) Buy Weed Without Breaking the Law

Congratulations! You live in a time when you can walk into a store and buy cannabis like it's a bag of Doritos. But before you do, let's talk about which states actually allow this.

Fully Legal States: The Land of the Free (Sort Of).

Some states have fully embraced cannabis, meaning you can buy, possess, and use it recreationally without fearing a SWAT team raid. These include places like California, Colorado, Oregon, and a growing list of chill states that realized they could make billions in tax revenue.

What you need to know:

- You must be 21+ to purchase recreational weed.
- You can buy from licensed dispensaries—not from your cousin's "business associate" who operates out of the alley behind the school and only takes cash because "banks can't be trusted."
- There are limits to how much you can buy and carry (usually around 1 ounce of flower or 8 grams of concentrate).
- No, you cannot smoke it anywhere you want—most states ban public consumption.

> *Pro Tip: If you're traveling, research local laws before you go—just because a state has legal cannabis doesn't mean you can smoke it wherever you want.*

Medical-Only States:
The "You Must Have a Note From Your Doctor" Club.

Other states allow medical marijuana only, meaning you need a doctor's approval and a medical card to buy legally. If you don't have one? Well, congratulations, you just committed a crime.

What you need to know:

- Qualifying conditions vary—some states only approve cannabis for things like epilepsy, while others are cool with anxiety and chronic pain.
- If you have a card, you can buy from licensed dispensaries, but it's still illegal for recreational use.
- If you don't have a card and buy from a dispensary anyway? Congratulations, you're now a criminal.

Totally Illegal States: The No-Fun Zones.

Then we have the states that still think cannabis is the Devil's Lettuce, where possessing even a little bit can land you in jail. These states include places like Idaho and Nebraska, where legislators still believe Reefer Madness was a documentary.

What you need to know:

- Having even a small amount can get you fined or arrested.
- There are no dispensaries, no medical programs, and no legal way to buy cannabis.
- Your best bet? Either move or invest in a really good lawyer.

How to Get Approved for Medical Marijuana: A Guide for the Medically Motivated

So, you live in a state where weed is still playing hard to get—recreational use is a no-go, but medical marijuana is allowed. Now, you're wondering, "How do I get approved?" and "Will I have to explain my entire medical history to a skeptical doctor who doesn't believe my back pain is *that* bad?"

Don't worry—I've got you covered. Here's everything you need to know about navigating the sometimes annoying, sometimes weird, but ultimately rewarding process of getting approved for medical cannabis.

Step 1: Check If You're Even Eligible (Do You Qualify to Join the Club?)

Before you start picking out your favorite strain, you need to figure out if your state thinks you deserve weed. Each state has its own list of qualifying conditions, which usually include:

- **Chronic pain** (because we all know, everyone over 30 qualifies)
- **Cancer** (because obviously)
- **Epilepsy or severe seizures**
- **Multiple sclerosis (MS)**
- **Glaucoma** (classic old-school reason)
- **PTSD** (in some states)
- **Crohn's disease or other severe gastrointestinal issues**
- **HIV/AIDS**
- **Severe nausea** (yes, this can be enough in some places)
- **Any terminal illness**

Some states let doctors approve anything they think qualifies (bless those states), while others have strict lists that leave you wondering why "being really stressed out" isn't on there.

How to Find Your State's Rules:

- Google: "Medical Marijuana Qualifying Conditions in [Your State]"
- Check your state's official Department of Health website (or just skim it for the important bits).
- Look for local dispensary websites—they usually break it down in plain English.

Step 2: Find a Doctor Who Won't Judge You.

Not all doctors are cool with medical cannabis. Some will give you the side-eye like you just asked for a prescription for a *kilo* of weed, while others will happily sign off because they *get it.*

What to Look For in a Doctor:

- A medical marijuana-friendly physician (Google "cannabis doctor near me" or use telehealth services).
- A doctor approved by your state's program (some states require special licensing).
- Someone who won't treat you like a criminal for asking about weed.

What to Expect in the Appointment:

- You'll explain your condition (translation: tell them how miserable you are).
- The doctor will ask about past treatments (yes, you can say "Nothing worked, and I want weed").
- If approved, they'll sign a certification that says you qualify for medical cannabis.

Pro Tip: Some states allow telemedicine, meaning you can get approved without even leaving your couch.

Step 3: Apply for Your Medical Marijuana Card
(The Fun Paperwork Part.)

If your doctor gives you the green light, you now have to apply through the state's official medical marijuana program. This usually involves:

- Filling out an application online
- Uploading your doctor's certification
- Providing proof of residency (usually a driver's license or utility bill)
- Paying a fee ($25 to $200, depending on the state and how much they want to rip you off)

Some states process applications fast (a few days), while others take their sweet time (weeks or months). Check processing times so you don't sit there wondering if they lost your paperwork.

Step 4: Visit a Dispensary
Like a Legitimate Cannabis Consumer.

Once your application is approved, you'll receive your medical marijuana card, and that's your golden ticket to the dispensary.

What You Need to Know About Shopping at a Dispensary:

- Bring your medical card and ID (yes, even if you look like a responsible adult).
- Expect limits on how much you can buy (states set different possession limits).
- Ask budtenders for advice—they're basically weed sommeliers.
- Prices may be lower for medical patients than for recreational users in states where both are legal.

Things to Watch Out For (or, Don't Mess This Up).

Expiration Dates Exist - Your medical marijuana card isn't forever. You'll need to renew it annually (which usually involves another doctor visit).

Not All Dispensaries Take Medical Cards from Other States - Some states recognize out-of-state medical cards (**hello, Oklahoma!**), but others don't. Check before you travel.

Employers Can Still Drug Test You - Some states protect medical users from being fired for cannabis use, but others don't. If your boss is anti-weed, be careful.

Federal Law is Still Stupid - Medical marijuana is legal in many states but still illegal federally. This means you can't fly with it, mail it, or take it onto federal property.

Is It Worth It?

If you live in a medical-only state, getting approved for a medical marijuana card is 100% worth the effort. You'll get access to:

- Stronger products.
- Better prices.
- Legal protection.

Just follow the steps, don't lose your card, and enjoy your new legally sanctioned cannabis experience. Now go forth and medicate responsibly!

> *Pro Tip: If you're buying CBD, look for labels that say "THC-Free" or "Broad-Spectrum" and check third-party lab results. Otherwise, you might end up getting fired over a gummy bear.*

Marijuana and Job Drug Testing: How to Keep Your Job and Your Sanity

So, weed is legal in your state, but guess what? That doesn't mean your job cares. In fact, many companies are still running their drug policies like it's 1995, testing for marijuana even when it's used off the clock. That leaves workers stuck in a weird gray area where what's legal isn't necessarily job-safe—kind of like how you *technically* can wear Crocs to a wedding, but should you? Probably not.

If you're trying to keep both your cannabis and your paycheck, here's what you need to know:

How Long Does THC Stay in Your System?

Unfortunately, weed doesn't just leave your body when the high wears off—it hangs around like an awkward houseguest who doesn't know when to leave. How long depends on:

- Your usage habits (occasional vs. daily smoker).
- Your metabolism (fast vs. slow).
- Your body fat percentage (THC is stored in fat).
- The type of test used (some tests are worse than others).

What Kind of Drug Tests Do Employers Use?

Most jobs don't care if you get high on your couch—they care if you're *high at work*. Unfortunately, drug tests don't measure impairment, just whether THC is somewhere in your system—even if it's been weeks. Here's what you might be up against for drug testing and how long they can detect THC:

1. Urine Test (Most Common) 3 to 30+ days (daily users, sorry—you're doomed for a while)

- Looks for THC metabolites (not active THC).

- Detects *past* use, not whether you're high at work.
- Used for pre-employment and random testing.

2. Saliva Test (Becoming More Popular) 24 to 48 hours (newer test, harder to cheat)

- Detects active THC, meaning it's looking for recent use.
- Harder to cheat (so don't even try that mouthwash trick).
- Used by law enforcement and some employers.

3. Blood Test (Rare but Scary) 1 to 2 days (unless you're a chronic user, then it's longer)

- Detects very recent use (*think within hours*).
- Used for accident investigations and DUIs.
- Unless you're in a wreck at work, you're probably safe.

4. Hair Follicle Test (The Worst One) (completely unnecessary, but some employers love suffering you the last 3 months.)

- Detects use up to 90 days back—because why not ruin your life?
- Used mainly for federal positions and very strict employers.

Key Takeaways:

- If you only *occasionally* partake, THC leaves your system faster.
- Daily smokers? Yeah... good luck passing a test any time soon.
- Hair tests are pure evil—but thankfully, not that common.

> *Pro Tip: If your job only does pre-employment testing, consider timing your fun accordingly. If they do random testing, welcome to the paranoia club.*

What Can You Take Without Testing Positive?

Not all cannabis products are created equal. Some will ruin your drug test, while others are safe for work (*assuming your boss doesn't mind CBD*).

✅ SAFE TO USE (Won't Trigger a Positive Test.)

- CBD Isolate – Pure CBD, zero THC.
- Broad-Spectrum CBD – Has multiple cannabinoids but no THC.

RISKY / WILL TEST POSITIVE.

- Full-Spectrum CBD – Contains up to 0.3% THC (yes, enough to fail).
- Delta-8, Delta-9, Delta-10 THC – Metabolizes into THC-COOH (in other words,.... you're busted).
- Hemp-Derived THC Products – Still has THC, which can accumulate.

Legal vs. Job Rules:
Is Testing for Weed the Same as Drinking on the Job?

Many companies still act like weed is some kind of dangerous voodoo, enforcing policies that don't match modern laws. But why do jobs test for marijuana and not alcohol?

The key difference lies in detection and workplace policies. Alcohol is legal nationwide, and its presence can be measured in real-time through a breathalyzer, which determines current impairment. As a result, most employers prohibit drinking on the job but have no issue with employees consuming alcohol on their own time.

In contrast, marijuana remains illegal at the federal level, even though many states have legalized it for medical or recreational use. Standard drug tests do not measure current impairment but instead detect THC metabolites, which can linger in the body for days or even weeks. This means an employee who smoked cannabis on their day off could still test positive long after the effects have worn off. Many workplaces enforce strict zero-tolerance policies for THC, banning its use entirely—even outside of work hours.

The reality is that while an employee can drink on a Saturday and show up Monday with no consequences, marijuana users risk failing a drug test simply for indulging on their personal time. Until workplace drug testing policies align with evolving cannabis laws, employees must continue navigating this unfair double standard.

How to Use Cannabis Without Getting Fired.

If you love both weed and employment, here's how to play it smart:

- Know your company's drug policy – Some don't test, others are strict.
- Understand your state's laws – Just because weed is legal doesn't mean your job allows it.
- Stick to THC-free products – If you must, CBD Isolate or Broad-Spectrum CBD is your best bet.
- Be cautious with Full-Spectrum CBD – Even legal hemp-based THC can build up in your system.

Until employers finally ditch outdated drug tests, using cannabis responsibly still comes with risks. Know the rules, be smart, and for the love of job security—don't get caught off guard by a surprise drug test.

> *Warning*: Found a website that promises "100% LEGAL WEED SHIPPED ANYWHERE"? Oh, go ahead and order—you might get some oregano, or maybe just a visit from the DEA.

Buying Weed Online:
Can You Actually Do This?

Short answer: **Not really.**

Longer answer: **Yes, but with major caveats.**

Legal Online Options.

If you live in a fully legal state, you can order weed online from a licensed dispensary, but you still have to pick it up or have it delivered by a licensed service (where allowed). Amazon is not going to start selling weed anytime soon.

Illegal Online Options
(How to End Up on a Government Watchlist.)

If you stumble upon a website offering to ship cannabis to any state, congratulations—you've found a scam or a felony in progress.

X Red Flags:

- "100% LEGAL WEED SHIPPED ANYWHERE IN THE USA" (No. Just... no.)
- Bitcoin-only payments (If you need crypto to buy it, you're probably funding something shady.)
- No license or business info on the website (Because they don't want to get caught, and neither should you.)

So, unless you enjoy dealing with dirt weed drugs, scammers, or federal agents, stick to legal dispensaries.

Traveling With Cannabis:
The Fastest Way to Ruin Your Vacation

Flying With Weed:
TSA's Favorite Game of "Will They Notice?"

So, you're about to hop on a plane and wondering, "Can I bring my weed with me?" The answer is: probably not a good idea.

Domestic Travel:

- TSA isn't actively looking for cannabis, but if they find it, they can report you to law enforcement.
- Some airports (like LAX) allow possession under state law, but once you leave the state, you might be breaking federal law.
- Edibles in an unmarked container? Probably fine.
- A whole-ass jar of weed? Maybe rethink that.

> *Pro Tip*: *Before traveling, consider buying what you need there unless you enjoy the thrill of asking airport security if they're "cool" with your stash.*

X International Travel:

- Do Not Do This.
- Many countries have zero tolerance for cannabis, meaning you could end up detained, fined, or worse.
- If you must bring anything, stick to CBD-only products (but even those are questionable in some places).

Driving Across State Lines:
Welcome to Federal Crime Land.

Even if cannabis is legal in both the state you're leaving *and* the one you're entering, taking it across state lines is a federal crime. That's right—crossing from California to Oregon with weed in your car is technically drug trafficking.

Risk Factors:

- Getting pulled over with out-of-state plates.
- Carrying more than the legal limit.
- Smelling like you just left a Snoop Dogg concert.

Moral of the story? Buy when you arrive, not before you leave.

Buying Weed for Someone Else:
Nice Gesture or Felony?

So, your elderly parent or anxious friend wants to try cannabis but doesn't know how to buy it. Can you buy it for them?

The Answer Depends:

- If they have a medical card: You might be able to purchase for them as a designated caregiver (depending on state laws).
- If it's recreational and they're 21+: You can buy it for them but giving them money to buy it themselves is safer.
- If they're underage or in an illegal state: Congratulations, you just committed drug distribution.

Moral of the story? Know the law before playing Weed Santa.

Legal State of Cannabis Today

Navigating the complex landscape of marijuana legalization in the United States can feel like trying to assemble IKEA furniture without the instructions. As of February 2025, the legal status of cannabis varies significantly across states, encompassing aspects such as medical use, recreational use, possession limits, cultivation rights, and product-specific regulations. Below is a comprehensive overview to help you understand the current state of marijuana laws in each state.

States with Legal Recreational and Medical Marijuana.

As of February 2025, 24 states and the District of Columbia have legalized both recreational and medical marijuana use.

In these states:

- Age Requirement: Adults aged 21 and over can purchase and possess cannabis.
- Possession Limits: Typically, individuals may possess up to 1–2 ounces of cannabis flower.
- Cultivation: Home cultivation is often permitted, with limits ranging from 4 to 12 plants per household.
- Product Regulations: Edibles, concentrates, and other cannabis-infused products are available, with THC content regulated to prevent excessively potent products.

Important: Crossing state lines with weed? Congrats, you're now a drug trafficker! The feds don't care that it's just a gummy. Leave it at home.

States with Medical Marijuana Only.

Thirty-nine states, three territories, and the District of Columbia have legalized medical marijuana as of February 2025.

In these jurisdictions:

- Qualifying Conditions: Patients with specific medical conditions (e.g., chronic pain, epilepsy) can obtain a medical marijuana card.
- Possession Limits: Patients are allowed to possess a certain amount, often up to a 30-day supply.
- Cultivation: Some states permit patients or caregivers to cultivate a limited number of plants.
- Product Regulations: There may be restrictions on THC content, especially for products accessible to minors.

States with Limited CBD/Low-THC Programs.

Several states have laws permitting the use of CBD oil or low-THC products, primarily for patients with specific medical conditions. These programs are more restrictive and do not allow the use of traditional cannabis products with higher THC levels.

States with No Legal Marijuana.

As of February 2025, 11 states have not legalized marijuana for medical or recreational use.

In these states:

- Possession: Any amount of marijuana possession is illegal and can result in criminal charges.
- Cultivation and Sale: Growing or selling marijuana is prohibited and subject to severe penalties.

Considerations for Non-Residents.

If you're traveling to a state where marijuana is legal:

- Purchasing: Non-residents can typically purchase cannabis, but there may be lower possession limits.

- Transporting: It's illegal to transport cannabis across state lines, even between states where it's legal.
- Consumption: Use is generally restricted to private residences; public consumption can lead to fines.

Product-Specific Regulations.

- Edibles: Many states cap the THC content per serving (commonly 5-10 mg) and per package to prevent overconsumption.
- Concentrates: Due to high potency, some states impose stricter possession limits on concentrates compared to flower.
- CBD Products: Hemp-derived CBD with less than 0.3% THC is federally legal, but state regulations can vary.

Staying Informed.

Marijuana laws are continually evolving. For the most current information:

- State Government Websites: Official state websites provide up-to-date legal information.
- Reputable Organizations: Groups like the National Conference of State Legislatures (NCSL) offer comprehensive resources. NCSL.ORG

Understanding the nuances of marijuana legalization in each state ensures responsible consumption and compliance with local laws. Always consult current state regulations before purchasing, possessing, or consuming cannabis products.

Cannabis Laws:
A Never-Ending Game of Whack-a-Mole

Cannabis laws are a mess—what's legal in one state is a felony in another, and federal law still treats it like heroin. The best way to not get arrested is to:

- Buy from licensed dispensaries only.
- Follow state laws—not just what your cousin told you.
- Never cross state lines with cannabis.
- Don't get too cocky—just because it's legal where you are doesn't mean you can light up anywhere.

Follow these simple guidelines, and you'll stay on the right side of the law—or at least out of serious trouble. Now that you know the legal dos and don'ts (and hopefully have a solid plan to avoid any awkward run-ins with law enforcement), it's time for the real adventure—finding the right dispensary.

Chapter 3:
How to Find the Right Dispensary (Without Looking Like a Lost Tourist)

So, you're ready to buy some legal weed, but now comes the real challenge: Where do you go, what do you ask, and how do you avoid looking like an undercover narc? Not all shops are created equal, and unless you enjoy overpaying for dry, bunk bud sold by someone who knows less than your grandma, you'll want to choose wisely.

Fear not—this guide will walk you through the essentials of dispensary shopping, So, let's break it down—where to go, what to look for, and how to walk out with exactly what you need (without looking like a total newbie).

Finding a Dispensary:
It's Not 2005 Anymore

Gone are the days when you had to rely on a shady guy named Vinny in a parking lot. Thanks to legalization, dispensaries are now Google-able, Yelp-reviewed, and even Instagram-verified. Here's how to find the best one:

Use Dispensary Locators.

Websites like:

- **Leafly** (leafly.com) – Like Yelp, but for weed.
- **Weedmaps** (weedmaps.com) – Shows menus, deals, and even customer reviews.
- **Google Maps** – Because some dispensaries don't advertise openly.

Check the Reviews (But Read Between the Lines).

- If you see "friendly staff" mentioned 50 times but nothing about the product quality, that's a red flag.
- If the reviews say, "prices are outrageous," believe them. Some dispensaries are basically Whole Foods but for weed.
- If someone mentions they got mysteriously "way too high" from a product, steer clear. That's code for bad labeling or inconsistent potency.

Look for Licensed Dispensaries.

You wouldn't buy sushi from a gas station (I hope), so don't buy weed from an unlicensed store. Most legal states have online databases where you can verify whether a dispensary is legit.

> *Important: A dispensary should feel like a pharmacy, not a back-alley black market. If the budtender says, "Uhhh, I think this one's good?" run.*

What to Ask Before You Buy

You don't need to sound like a weed scholar, but a little knowledge goes a long way. Here are some key questions:

"What's your most popular product for [sleep/anxiety/pain/fun]?"

Dispensary staff ("budtenders") love helping people find the right product. Just don't be vague—saying "I want weed" is like walking into a bar and saying, "I want alcohol."

"What's the difference between these strains?"

If they can't explain the difference between indica, sativa, and hybrid, find another dispensary.

"Do you have any first-time buyer discounts?"

Many dispensaries offer huge discounts for first-time customers—sometimes up to 30% off or free pre-rolls.

"How potent is this?"

- Flower: Measured in THC percentage (10–30% is common).
- Edibles: Measured in milligrams of THC (start with 5mg, or less for first timers, unless you enjoy existential crises).
- Concentrates: Measured in fear and regret (often 70%+ THC).

"Do you have the full COA (Certificate of Analysis)?"

Ask for the lab testing certificate and scrutinize it like a stoner checking their bag for missing nugs. Look for red flags, missing data, or numbers that seem too good to be true.

"Do I need cash?"

Most dispensaries are cash-only due to federal banking laws. Some have ATMs, but they charge fees that would make an airport blush.

What Even Is a Cannabis Testing Lab?
The Wild West of Weed Science

Ah, the modern marvel of independent cannabis testing labs—those gleaming temples of science where white-coated professionals use cutting-edge equipment to ensure your weed isn't just sawdust and false hope. At least, that's the dream. The reality? Well, let's just say if you thought the cannabis industry was a well-regulated, buttoned-up affair, I've got a bridge in Colorado to sell you (THC-infused, of course).

In theory, these labs exist to protect consumers by analyzing THC and CBD content, screening for contaminants, and making sure your pricey eighth isn't 60% oregano. They're supposed to test for pesticides, mold, heavy metals, and residual solvents—things you don't want in your lungs unless you're into huffing lead paint for fun.

But here's the catch: cannabis testing is like the Wild West of science. Labs operate under a patchwork of state laws, private accreditation, and industry "standards" that often have the consistency of a gas-station pre-roll. The result? A system where one lab's 30% THC super-strain might test at 18% in another lab... or 42% in a lab that's been "friendly" to growers with deep pockets.

> **Warning**: If your budtender can't explain what they're selling, they're either high or incompetent—either way, this isn't where you want to make your first purchase.

Can You Actually Trust What the Labs Say?

Short answer: Maybe.

Long answer: Only if you know what to look for.

Many testing labs are legitimate and follow good practices, but let's be real—some are glorified rubber stamps for growers looking to market their "face-meltingly potent" strain at a premium price. Here's how to spot the difference:

Accreditation Matters (Sort Of).

A real, science-driven lab should be ISO/IEC 17025 accredited. This means they meet international standards for laboratory competence.

If a lab can't show accreditation—or claims their "buddy who's great at chemistry" handles testing—run.

Check the Lab's Reputation.

Look up reviews. If customers repeatedly say a lab's test results are inconsistent, that's a red flag.

Watch for labs that magically produce high THC numbers every time. Cannabis growers love a lab that "somehow" always finds their flower tests at 35% THC.

See If They Provide Full COAs (Certificates of Analysis).

A legit lab report should show not just THC/CBD levels, but also pesticide levels, microbial contamination, heavy metals, and residual solvents.

If all you're seeing is a THC number in big, bold letters, you're probably looking at a marketing tool, not a scientific report.

Do the THC Numbers Pass the Smell Test?

If a strain claims to be 40% THC, congratulations, you've found either the strongest cannabis known to man or a lab that needs to put down the bong and recalibrate its equipment.

Most high-quality flower maxes out around 25-30% THC. If someone's consistently hitting numbers beyond that, there's a very good chance they're paying for inflated results.

What's Legally Required?

The rules depend on the state. Some states (like Colorado and California) require testing for potency and contaminants before a product hits dispensary shelves. Others have looser regulations, letting producers essentially self-report numbers. Because nothing says "trustworthy" like letting the seller grade their own homework.

Even in states with solid testing laws, enforcement is often a joke. Labs have been caught tweaking results, inflating THC percentages to help growers market their products, or outright faking results to keep clients happy. After all, if a lab gets a reputation for "low" THC numbers, producers will just take their business to a friendlier competitor.

What Does This Mean for You?

If you're buying legal cannabis, don't just assume the THC number on the package is gospel. Look for dispensaries that work with reputable labs, check COAs if they're available, and trust your own experience over flashy numbers. A well-grown, 20% THC strain can hit just as hard as an artificially inflated "35%" strain that's been blessed by a questionable lab.

And if you're buying from a shady source? Well, let's just say your testing options are limited to the ancient art of "smoking it and seeing what happens."

> *Pro Tip: Always buy from legit sources. If someone offers you a "really good deal" on weed from the trunk of their car, walk away.*

How to Read a COA (Certificate of Analysis) Without Feeling Like You Need a Science Degree

So, you've finally decided to be a responsible cannabis connoisseur and check out a COA (Certificate of Analysis) before buying your bud. Good for you! Unfortunately, reading one of these things can sometimes feel like deciphering an ancient scroll—except instead of hidden treasure, you're trying to figure out whether your weed is legit or laced with pesticides.

A COA is the lab report that breaks down what's actually in your cannabis. Dispensaries and growers (at least in legal markets) are supposed to have these available for customers. If they don't? That's already a red flag. But assuming they do, let's go over what a typical COA should show and how to read one without getting scammed. What's on a COA?

A legitimate COA should include the following key sections:

1. **Product Information & Lab Details**. This is the "official" section where you'll see:

- The name of the lab that tested the product.
- The date of testing (because old results are useless).
- The batch number (to track which crop this came from).
- The strain name or product type (flower, concentrate, edible, etc.)

X Red Flags:

- No lab name?
- No batch number?
- Run. This is like getting a mystery bottle of pills with no label.

2. **Cannabinoid Profile** (THC, CBD, and Friends)

This is what most people obsess over—the THC and CBD percentages—but it's just one part of the story. A good COA will show:

- THC (Δ9-THC & THCA) – The total THC content, with THCA being the raw form that turns into THC when heated.
- CBD (CBD & CBDA) – Same deal—CBDA converts into CBD when smoked/vaped.
- Other Cannabinoids (CBG, CBN, CBC, etc.) – These play supporting roles in your high.

✗ Red Flags:

- No breakdown between THCA and Δ9-THC? This means you're not seeing the full picture of how potent the weed will be after smoking.
- Inflated THC numbers (e.g., 40%+ THC flower) – Someone's lying, and it's not the science.

3. **Terpene Profile** (What Actually Determines Your High)

If the lab is legit, the COA will include a terpene breakdown, which tells you what kind of experience to expect:

- Limonene – Uplifting, citrusy, anti-anxiety.
- Myrcene – Sedating, couch-lock, earthy.
- Pinene – Focused, pine-scented, alertness booster.
- Caryophyllene – Stress relief, spicy aroma.

✗ Red Flags:

- No terpene data? It might not be required, but if a grower wants to prove quality, they'll include it.

4. **Contaminant Testing** (Because You Don't Want to Smoke Poison)

This is where things get serious. Good labs will test for:

- Pesticides – Because inhaling bug spray is bad for you.
- Heavy Metals – Lead, arsenic, and mercury have no place in your lungs.
- Residual Solvents – If it's a concentrate, they check for leftover chemicals from extraction.
- Microbial Contaminants – Mold, mildew, and other nasties that should never be in your weed.

✗ Red Flags:

- No contaminants section? Major red flag. Any legitimate lab test will confirm the product is safe to consume.

How to Use a COA to Make Smart Choices

- Don't Just Look at THC – Check the terpenes to predict how the high will feel.
- Check for Contaminants – Make sure you're not inhaling pesticides or mold.
- Verify the Lab – If you're suspicious, Google the lab name. If they don't have a real website or reviews, the results might be fake.

Demand a COA, or Walk Away

A proper COA isn't just a piece of paper—it's proof that what you're smoking is safe and accurately labeled. If a dispensary won't show you the COA, they either don't have one, or they don't want you to see it. Either way, that's not a place you want to buy from. Because if you're paying top dollar for "premium" cannabis, the least they can do is prove it isn't filled with mold, lead, and lies.

Example of a COA Breakdown
(What You'll Actually See on One)

Here's a simplified example of a COA you might find in a dispensary:

- Product Name: Super Chill OG
- Batch Number: SC-420-0325
- Lab Name: Honest Bud Testing Inc.
- Test Date: 02/25/2025

Cannabinoid Profile
- THCA: 24.1%
- Δ9-THC: 2.1%
- Total THC (after conversion): 22.5%
- CBDA: 0.2%
- Total CBD: 0.1%
- CBG: 1.2%

Terpene Profile
- Limonene: 0.8%
- Myrcene: 1.5%
- Caryophyllene: 0.9%

Contaminant Testing
- Pesticides: PASS
- Heavy Metals: PASS
- Microbial Contaminants: PASS

Pro Tip: Many dispensaries offer first-time buyer discounts. So yes, being an overanxious newbie actually saves you money for once!

How Much Can You Buy and Possess?

Each state has its own laws because nothing about cannabis is ever simple. Generally speaking, legal limits apply to both purchases and possession—so just because you can *buy* a certain amount doesn't mean you can *carry* that much without breaking the law.

General Guidelines (Subject to State Laws):

- Flower (the actual buds): Usually 1–2 ounces per day for recreational users.
- Edibles: Typically, 100mg–800mg of THC total (so don't expect to walk out with a Costco-sized tub of gummies).
- Concentrates (wax, shatter, oils): Usually 5–8 grams.
- CBD Products: Often unlimited (because nobody's getting arrested for lotion).

Can You Buy More in a Single Day by Going to Multiple Dispensaries?

Technically, yes—dispensaries don't share real-time data (yet). But if you get caught with too much, good luck explaining why you're carrying enough weed to tranquilize a horse.

What About Medical Users?

If you have a medical card, you usually get:

- Higher possession limits
- Stronger products
- Lower taxes (which is the real win here)

Buying Weed as an Out-of-State Visitor: Proceed with Caution

Traveling to a legal state and planning to stock up? Read this carefully before you make a very dumb mistake.

Can You Buy Weed If You're Not a Resident?

Yes—most legal states allow non-residents to purchase cannabis. However:

- Some states have lower purchase limits for non-residents (Colorado, for example, limits you to half an ounce instead of a full ounce).
- You still need to be 21+ (unless you have a medical card).

Can You Take It Home?

Absolutely not. (Unless you like committing federal crimes.)

- Flying with weed: TSA doesn't actively search for cannabis, but if they find it, they can refer it to local law enforcement. If you're lucky, they'll just throw it away. If you're *unlucky*, congratulations—you just made your flight much more expensive.
- Driving across state lines: Even if both states have legal weed, crossing state lines with it is illegal. Yes, even if you're going from California to Oregon.

Can You Mail It to Yourself?

No. Stop it. Don't even think about it. Mailing weed is a federal offense, and unless you're looking for a starring role on *Cops: Special Cannabis Edition*, it's a terrible idea.

Now Venture Forth and Buy:
Dispensary Shopping Like a Pro

Buying legal weed should be as easy as buying groceries, but thanks to ridiculous laws, it's still more complicated than it needs to be. Here's how to make it smooth:

- Find a reputable dispensary using Weedmaps, Leafly, or Google reviews.
- Ask the right questions about potency, first-time discounts, and payment methods.
- Know your purchase limits (especially as an out-of-state visitor).
- Never, ever, EVER try to fly or drive across state lines with weed.

Follow these tips, and you'll look like a seasoned pro instead of an overwhelmed tourist. Now go forth, buy wisely, and please—don't be the person who asks if they can "just get a single joint." They'll laugh at you.

In the next section, we'll get into the fun part—how to actually consume cannabis without looking like a total amateur. So, stay tuned, and maybe grab a snack. You're going to need it.

Pro Tip: If you get too high and feel like your soul is leaving your body, relax—nobody has ever died from weed. Drink some water, put on cartoons, and accept that time is now meaningless.

Chapter 4: How to Actually Use This Stuff Without Embarrassing Yourself (or Dying of Anxiety)

So, you've legally (hopefully) acquired some cannabis. Congratulations! You're now the proud owner of a plant that has been used for thousands of years, demonized for about a hundred, and is now slowly being accepted again because the government realized they could tax the hell out of it.

But now comes the real challenge: How do you actually use it without coughing up a lung, greening out, or ending up so high that you start texting your ex about "energy vibrations"?

So, you've learned the basics—what cannabis is, how it works, and that your body was basically built for it (seriously, scientists say so). You have learned how, what and where to purchase and now comes the fun part: figuring out how to actually consume it without turning yourself into a cautionary tale.

Let's talk logistics. You wouldn't shotgun tequila alone in an alley, would you? (If you would, please seek help, but not from me). Same rules apply here. Your first time getting high should be in a safe, controlled environment—not in the middle of Walmart at 2 a.m. with a cart full of frozen pizzas. Find a trusted, sober buddy—your 'wingman' in this grand adventure. Their job? To remind you that time isn't actually stopping and that no, your hands are not getting smaller. They will also be the hero who ensures you don't decide to text your ex or start a philosophical debate with your cat.

Long gone are the days when smoking a joint was your only option. Today, cannabis comes in more forms than Starbucks drinks, each with its own effects, onset time, and likelihood of making you text your ex. Let's break them down so you can make informed choices—rather than just grabbing whatever looks the coolest at the dispensary and hoping for the best.

This chapter will guide you through the fine art of consuming cannabis like a responsible, semi-functional adult—instead of a college freshman who just ate an entire weed brownie because "it wasn't kicking in."

But first let's talk about health concerns for contraindications & precautions. What not to do (unless you like living on the edge).

Avoiding Disasters with your Health: Because Who Needs More Chaos?

Alright, before you light up, pop an edible, or dive headfirst into the dispensary menu, let's have a little chat about who might need to pump the brakes—or at least proceed with caution. I am not a doctor and this is not health advice. Just like alcohol, caffeine, or signing up for a gym membership you'll never use, cannabis isn't for everyone in every situation. There are some cases where you need to think twice, consult a pro (Yes, there are professional cannabis guides), or at the very least, not be an idiot about it.

1. Pregnancy & Lactation: No, the Baby Doesn't Need a Contact High.

Look, if you're pregnant or nursing, this isn't just about you anymore—there's a tiny human involved. The research on cannabis use during pregnancy is still murky, but some studies suggest it might affect fetal development, leading to low birth weight, preterm labor, or potential neurodevelopmental effects. And since THC can pass through breast milk, your newborn might end up with their first high way before their first steps—which is not ideal. Until we know more, the general advice is just don't (and if you're considering it for medical reasons, talk to an actual doctor, not your 'holistic' cousin Harmony).

2. Family History of Psychosis or Schizophrenia: This One's Important.

If your family tree has branches of psychosis or schizophrenia, cannabis—especially high-THC strains—might not be your friend. Some studies suggest that heavy cannabis use could increase the risk of triggering or worsening symptoms in those already genetically predisposed. Does this mean one puff is going to send you into a psychotic break? No. But if mental health conditions run in your family, proceed with caution, opt for lower-THC strains, or consider CBD-only options (and, again, maybe run this by a mental health professional who actually knows your history).

3. Kids & Teens: Let's Not Fry Developing Brains.

You wouldn't hand a 12-year-old a beer and tell them to 'enjoy responsibly,' right? Same logic applies here. The teen brain is still under construction, and regular cannabis use before age 25 could affect memory, learning, and impulse control (which, let's face it, teenagers are already struggling with). This doesn't mean cannabis is evil—it just means that if you're underage (21 in most states), it's best to wait until your brain is fully built before experimenting. Future You will thank you.

4. Lung Issues (COPD & Asthma): Maybe Skip the Smoke.

If your lungs already have a hard time dealing with oxygen, adding smoke or vapor into the mix is probably not the best plan. Smoking anything—weed, tobacco, or that questionable incense your roommate insists 'clears energy'—can irritate the lungs. If you have asthma or COPD (Chronic Obstructive Pulmonary Disease), consider non-inhaled options like edibles, tinctures, or topicals. You don't have to suffer through a wheezing fit just to get the benefits.

5. Substance Use Disorder: Know Your Addictions.

If you've struggled with addiction in the past (or present), it's worth pausing to consider how cannabis fits into your life. While many people use cannabis as an exit drug—helping them move away from alcohol, opioids, or other substances—some may find it triggers addictive patterns. Cannabis can be habit-forming especially if it becomes a coping mechanism instead of a mindful choice. This doesn't mean you're out, but you should talk with a professional who won't just say 'bro, you'll be fine.'

Bonus: Drug Interactions: Because Mixing Stuff Can Get Weird

Cannabis might be natural, but that doesn't mean it plays nice with everything in your medicine cabinet. It can interact with blood thinners, sedatives, antidepressants, and certain heart medications—sometimes making them stronger or weaker than they should be. If you're on medication, check with a professional before you find yourself wondering why your usual dose of Xanax suddenly feels like a tranquilizer dart. Be safe—Google is not a doctor.

None of this means you can't use cannabis—it just means you might need a game plan. If you fall into any of these categories, work with a medical professional, choose products wisely, and always listen to your body. Cannabis can be a great tool, but like power tools, tequila, or group chats with 20+ people—it's best used responsibly. Now, it's time to learn how to use this magic "Bud".

Smoking:
The Classic Fastest Way to Announce to Everyone That You're High

Ah, smoking—the timeless tradition of rolling up some green, lighting it on fire, and inhaling like you're in a Cheech and Chong movie. Smoking cannabis is the oldest and most obvious method, and it's also the one that will immediately make you smell like a reggae festival. If you think of cannabis, this is probably the first method that comes to mind. And while it's definitely effective, it's not for everyone.

If you go this route, you'll need to decide how you want to smoke. Options include joints (the rolled-up kind), blunts (the bigger, tobacco-wrapped kind), and pipes (for those who want to feel like an old-timey wizard). Each has its own vibe, but ultimately, it's just different ways to burn the same plant.

Your Options:

- **Joints** – Basically a weed cigarette. Easy to roll (for some), burns quickly, and perfect for sharing, assuming you like swapping saliva with friends.
- **Blunts** – Like a joint but bigger and wrapped in tobacco leaf, because nothing says "health-conscious" like mixing cannabis with nicotine.
- **Pipes** – Great for those who don't want to waste time rolling. Just pack, light, and wonder why you suddenly forgot what day it is.
- **Bongs** – For those who want to take one hit and immediately cross over into that surreal alternate universe (Happy Place).

✅ Pros of Smoking:

- Fast-acting - You'll feel the effects within minutes. No waiting around wondering if you took enough.

- Control - You can take a little, see how you feel, and adjust accordingly. Easy to dose—just stop when you feel good (or start panicking).
- No mystery ingredients - Just pure flower—no weird additives. Classic and nostalgic, like your grandpa's old war stories but less depressing.

✗ Cons of Smoking:

- Harsh on the lungs - If you enjoy hacking up a lung, you'll love it. If you're new to smoking, expect coughing. A lot of coughing.
- Smell - Your clothes, your hair, your entire house—everything will smell like a reggae concert. You will smell like weed. Forever. Even if you shower.
- Not subtle - You can't really light up at a family gathering and expect no one to notice. People will know. Even your nosy neighbor Karen.

> *Important: Start low and slow. You wouldn't chug an entire bottle of tequila on your first drink (hopefully), so don't inhale half a blunt thinking you'll "just see how it goes."*

Bong vs. Pipe:
The Great Debate in Getting High

So, you've decided to step up from rolling joints like an amateur and are now faced with a crucial decision—bong or pipe? While both serve the same noble purpose (getting you gloriously high), they do so in very different ways, each with their own perks, pitfalls, and potential for embarrassing yourself.

The Bong: A Water-Fueled Thrill Ride.

Bongs use water filtration to cool and smooth out the smoke before it hits your throat and lungs. This means less coughing, fewer regretful hacking fits, and a more enjoyable smoking experience. But before you get too excited, keep in mind that this filtration can also remove some cannabinoids and terpenes, meaning you might not get the full flavor and intensity compared to a pipe.

✅ Pros of a Bong:

- Smoother Hits – The water cools down the smoke, making it gentler on your throat.
- Bigger Rips – With one deep inhale, you can take in more smoke than you ever intended.
- Filters Out Some Toxins – The water traps ash and some combustion byproducts. (Science!)

✗ Cons of a Bong:

- Not Exactly Portable – Try stuffing one in your pocket. (Or don't.)
- Breakable – Glass bongs don't bounce. They shatter, usually at the worst possible time.
- Harder to Clean – Ever smelled stale bong water? Exactly.

Buying a Bong: Welcome to the Glass Jungle

Thinking of investing in a bong? Get ready for some choices. A small one is portable (ish), but a big one might deliver a hit so intense you forget your name—and maybe your address. Don't just buy the tallest thing in the store because it looks like a science project. Bigger isn't always better unless you're training for the Cannabis Olympics.

Most bongs are made of glass (great flavor, easy to break) or plastic (less glamorous, more forgiving). Some have percolators and ice catchers—which sound fancy, but mostly just add cleaning steps and more ways to break things.

Buy something that matches your lifestyle. If you're clumsy, forgetful, or hate cleaning anything more complicated than a coffee mug, keep it simple. If you're into bubble-filled, slow-mo cinematic rips, go wild—but maybe take out insurance.

The Pipe: Simple, Reliable, Harsh.

Pipes are small, discreet, and require no setup, making them the Swiss Army knife of weed consumption. However, they come with a major downside: zero filtration. Every hit is unfiltered, meaning it's hot, harsh, and full of every little bit of burnt plant matter you probably didn't need in your lungs.

✓ Pros of a Pipe:

- Portable – Toss it in your pocket and you're ready to go.
- No Setup Required – Just load, light, and inhale.
- Durable (Sometimes) – Metal and silicone pipes can survive the apocalypse.

✗ Cons of a Pipe:

- Harsh on the Throat and Lungs – Be prepared to cough like you just ran a marathon.
- Hot Smoke – There's no water to cool it down before it scorches your lungs.
- Less Filtration = More Toxins – You're getting all the good stuff...and all the bad stuff.

Picking the Right Pipe: Not Just a Tiny Bowl on a Stick

So you're buying a pipe—great! Now prepare to overthink it. Pipes come in more shapes and sizes than you'd expect. Chillums are tiny and stealthy but hit like you're sipping fire through a coffee straw. Sherlock pipes look cool and deliver smoother hits, but suddenly you're packing a pipe that needs its own travel case.

Pay attention to the bowl size—a wide bowl is great for quick solo hits; a deeper one works for longer sessions or sharing. And don't sleep on the little features:

- A carb hole helps control airflow (aka not coughing up your soul)
- A screen prevents burning ash from blasting straight into your lungs (unless you like surprises)
- Stem length affects heat—longer = cooler smoke

Metal pipes are durable and taste like nickels. Glass pipes are flavorful and break if you breathe near them wrong. Wood pipes are classy, but taste like your old coffee mug. Choose your pipe like you'd choose a roommate: dependable, low-drama, and unlikely to give you second-degree burns.

The Absorption & Intensity Factor: Which Gets You Higher?

A bong's cooler, smoother hits allow you to take in more smoke at once, which often leads to a faster, more intense high compared to a pipe. However, because the water filters out some compounds, the high may feel slightly "cleaner" but a bit less flavorful. Pipes, on the other hand, hit harder and faster since nothing is getting filtered out, but you might cough up half your lung in the process.

Alternative Bong Liquids: Because Water is Too Mainstream

Now, let's talk about the wild idea of swapping out that boring old H_2O for something...more exciting. (Spoiler alert: some of these are great, and some are absolutely terrible ideas.)

Water – The Classic Choice.

- Effect: Clean, smooth, and reliable.
- Flavor: Neutral. Doesn't mess with your weed's taste.
- Verdict: The gold standard for a reason.

Champagne – The Fancy Experiment.

- Effect: The carbonation makes the smoke *tingle* a bit.
- Flavor: Slightly sweet and bubbly—until it goes flat and gross.
- Verdict: Fun for a party trick but stick to drinking it.

Snow – The Frosty Treat.

- Effect: Super chilled hits that feel smooth and refreshing.
- Flavor: Neutral, but colder than your ex's heart.
- Verdict: A+ for smoothness, but annoying to constantly replace.

X Alcohol – The Terrible Idea.

- Effect: Burns like hell. Absorbs THC, meaning you're losing potency.
- Flavor: Straight regret.
- Verdict: **DO NOT DO THIS**. Unless you enjoy inhaling fire.

So, which is it for you? Bong or Pipe?

If you want a smoother, more enjoyable experience, go with a bong. If you need something quick, simple, and portable, grab a pipe. Just don't use alcohol in your bong, unless you enjoy the feeling of inhaling a demon's breath. Either way, start slow—because "too high" is a real place, and it's not fun.

> *Warning*: Just because it's legal in some states doesn't mean you can light up in the middle of a Starbucks. Know the laws before you become an accidental activist.

Vaping: The Fancy, Futuristic, and Probably-Healthier Option (Maybe?)

Vaping is the modern, sleek, slightly suspicious cousin of smoking. Instead of burning the plant, vapes heat cannabis just enough to release its active compounds as vapor—hence the name. Vaping is the sleek version of smoking weed. No rolling, no lighter—just press a button and inhale like you're in a sci-fi movie.

Types of Vapes:

- Oil Pens - Portable, discreet, and easy to overuse because they hit so smoothly.
- Dry Herb Vaporizers - Heat the flower without burning it, which is great for flavor nerds and people who hate coughing.

✅ Pros of Vaping:

- Discreet - No lingering smell, no giant cloud of smoke, easy to carry, and no need to explain yourself to nosy neighbors.
- Less harsh - No burning means no throat on fire. Easier on the lungs than smoking.
- Instant effects without the long-term regret of edibles.
- Portability - Vape pens fit right in your pocket and look like regular e-cigarettes, making it easier to avoid judgmental stares.

✗ Cons of Vaping:

- Not all vapes are created equal - Vape cartridges can be cut with unknown goo. Some contain questionable additives, so buy from reputable sources unless you enjoy chemical roulette gambling with your lungs.
- Can sneak up on you - The high feels smoother, so it's easy to overdo it without realizing. You will puff on it constantly because it's too easy.

- Expensive - Good vapes are not cheap.
- Battery dependency - Nothing kills the vibe like a dead vape pen. Charge that thing.

If you go this route, make sure you're getting high-quality oil or flower—not the cheapest vape cart you can find at a gas station. No one wants to be the person who "just wanted to relax" but ended up on a three-hour existential crisis because their vape was laced with mystery chemicals.

Edibles:
The "Oh No, I Took Too Much" Category

Edibles seem innocent enough—after all, they're just tasty treats infused with cannabis. But make no mistake: these little bastards will ruin you if you're not careful. If you've heard one horror story about cannabis, it probably involves edibles. Someone eats a cookie, feels nothing after 20 minutes, eats another, and then suddenly their soul leaves their body.

Edibles are awesome—but also deceptive. Since they have to go through your digestive system, they take longer to kick in. And when they do, they tend to hit harder and last longer than smoking or vaping.

How Edibles Work:

Listen up, future edible enthusiast—if you're about to pop a THC gummy on an empty stomach, you're doing it wrong. Cannabis is lipophilic, which is a fancy science word for 'it loves fat'—kind of like how you love fries at 2 a.m. after a long night of partying. When you eat cannabis, it goes through your liver, which transforms THC into a stronger compound that hits harder and lasts longer. Translation? You will be high for HOURS.

This means that THC and CBD absorb better when consumed with a little dietary fat, so do yourself a favor and have a snack. A burger? Great. Some avocado toast? Sure, be that person. A spoonful of peanut butter like a feral raccoon? Even better. The point is, eating something will help your body actually use the THC instead of sending it straight to the void. Plus, let's be real—having snacks before the munchies hit is just solid life planning.

When it comes to edibles, starting small is never a bad idea—seriously, we're talking 1mg. Better safe than sorry, right? Many newcomers dive in with a "more is better" mindset, but the truth is, it's way easier to adjust upwards than to ride out an accidental overindulgence. So, go ahead and take baby steps. Start low, and give it time to kick in—remember, edibles take longer to hit, so patience is key. If you don't feel it maybe try more next time (like at least a day, not 30 minutes later).

Golden Rules of Edibles:

- Start Low, Go Slow. If the package says 5mg is a serving, don't eat 50mg just because you "don't feel anything yet."
- Wait at least 90 minutes before taking more. The number of people who have eaten a second brownie and ended up talking to their furniture is astronomical.
- Know your dosage. Anything over 10mg is for pros—if you're new, 1mg is okay to be sure. 2.5-5mg is plenty unless you enjoy seeing through time.

✅ Pros of Edibles:

- No smoking required - Perfect for people who don't want to inhale anything. No smoke, no smell—your neighbor Karen won't know.
- Longer-lasting high - Great for sustained relief but also means you're in it for the long haul. It lasts way longer (4-8 hours or more).

- Tasty options - Gummies, chocolates, cookies, even drinks — like a candy store, but more fun.

✗ Cons of Edibles:

- The waiting game - Effects can take 30 minutes to 2 hours to show up, leading impatient people to make terrible decisions. Takes forever to kick in, leading to the classic "I don't feel it yet" mistake.
- Harder to dose - Once it's in your system, you can't undo it. No "let me just smoke a little less" option here. If you overdo it, you're stuck for hours—there's no turning back.
- Potency varies - One brand's "mild" edible might send you to another dimension. Always start low and slow—5mg of THC is a good beginner dose. Take too much and you will forget what "normal" feels like.

If you try edibles, read the packaging carefully. A single cookie might actually be four servings, so unless you want to astral project to another plane of existence, don't eat the whole thing at once.

> *Warning*: Edibles are not instant. If you don't feel anything after 30 minutes, DO NOT eat more. Unless you want to spend the next six hours questioning reality and sweating.

THC-Infused Drinks: What You Need to Know

So, you've decided to explore the world of THC-infused drinks. Good for you! Maybe you're looking for a new way to relax without smoking, or perhaps you just enjoy the idea of getting a buzz from something that tastes like a fancy craft beverage instead of burnt leaves. Either way, welcome to the THC drink universe—where the effects can be smooth and enjoyable or sneak up on you like a raccoon rifling through your trash at 2 AM.

Different Types of THC Drinks.

First things first: not all THC drinks are created equal. Some are hemp-derived, meaning they contain no more than 0.3% Delta-9 THC by dry weight, making them federally legal but still capable of producing a high. Others are marijuana-derived, which means they contain more than 0.3% THC and are only available in states where cannabis is legal. Then there are CBD-infused drinks that won't get you high but might help you relax, and THC + CBD combination drinks that offer a balanced effect, depending on the ratio.

- **Hemp-Derived THC Drinks** (≤0.3% Delta-9 THC): Legal in most states, can still produce a mild high.
- **Marijuana-Derived THC Drinks** (>0.3% Delta-9 THC): Available only in legal states, generally more potent.
- **CBD-Infused Drinks**: No high, just relaxation.
- **THC + CBD Combo Drinks**: Balanced effects, with varying THC-to-CBD ratios.

How to Read Labels & Not Accidentally Drink a Mistake.

Yes, I know you're excited but pause for a second and check what's in this thing. Before cracking open that bottle of bliss, take a second to read the label—seriously, do it. You need to check how much THC is in it per serving, because many drinks contain multiple servings, and you don't want to learn that lesson the hard way. Don't assume it's a single serving unless you enjoy spontaneous naps in inconvenient places. That entire drink may have enough THC to make your couch feel like a spaceship.

Are you sipping a mild 2.5 mg THC spritzer, or did you just crack open a 100 mg bottle of regret? The difference is significant.

A bottle might look like a single-serving delight, but it could be packing enough THC to turn your casual Tuesday night into a deep philosophical debate with your teddy bear.

Also, keep an eye out for the type of THC used. Is it Delta-9, Delta-8, Delta-10, or some wildcard like THC-O? Delta-9 is your classic high, Delta-8 is a bit more mellow, and Delta-10 is said to be more uplifting and social. THC-O? Well, let's just say you might want to sit down for that one.

Another important thing to note is whether the THC is nano-emulsified. If it is, that means it'll kick in faster (around 15-30 minutes), whereas traditional THC drinks can take 45-90 minutes. This is crucial information because impatience is the number one reason people accidentally overdo it. Here is what you should look for:

- **THC Content**: Listed in milligrams (mg) per serving and per container.
- **Serving Size**: The whole bottle may not be one serving—check before chugging!
- **Type of THC**: Delta-9, Delta-8, Delta-10, or synthetic versions like THC-O.
- **Onset Time**: Regular THC drinks take 45-90 minutes; nano-emulsified versions kick in within 15-30 minutes.
- **Additional Ingredients**: Look for sugar, caffeine, alcohol, or adaptogens.
- **Lab Testing (COA)**: Always check for third-party testing to verify THC content and purity.

How Strong is Too Strong?

Let's talk potency. If you're new to this, start with 2.5-5 mg of THC. That'll give you a mild buzz without turning your night into a psychedelic circus. If you have some experience, 5-10 mg is a solid choice for noticeable but manageable effects. Anything above 10 mg is for those who know exactly what they're doing, and beyond

20 mg? Well, let's just say you might want to clear your schedule and prepare for deep thoughts about why giraffes have such long necks.

✅ Pros of THC infused drinks:

- Discreet & Smoke-Free – No need to reek of weed or fumble with rolling papers. Just sip and enjoy.
- Precise Dosing – Unlike homemade edibles, you know exactly how much THC you're consuming.
- Longer-Lasting Effects – Compared to smoking, the high lasts longer, making it great for extended relaxation.
- Tastes Better Than a Joint – Many THC drinks are crafted to taste like cocktails or sodas, so you're not inhaling something that tastes like your lawn.
- No Lung Irritation – Perfect for those who want to avoid coughing fits or explaining why their voice suddenly sounds like a blues singer.

❌ Cons of THC infused drinks:

- Takes Longer to Kick In – If you're impatient, you might be tempted to drink more before the first dose hits. That's how people end up too high to function.
- Can Be Overpowering – If you misjudge the dose, you may find yourself glued to your couch questioning your cat about where it hid the munchies.
- Serving Sizes Can Be Misleading – Just because it's one can doesn't mean it's one serving. Read the fine print before you go full send.
- Harder to Control the High – Unlike smoking, where the effects wear off quicker, a THC drink high can last for hours, so cancel any immediate responsibilities.
- Crossfading Can Get Messy – Drinking alcohol with THC can amplify both effects, often leading to nausea, dizziness, and regret.

How to Use THC Drinks Without Regrets.

So, you've decided to go the classy route and drink your THC instead of puffing it out of a poorly rolled joint like a college freshman. Good choice—probably. THC drinks can be smooth, enjoyable, and discreet. They can also creep up on you like that coworker who swears they're "just having one drink" but ends up singing karaoke on a table an hour later. Alright, let's go over the basics so you don't end up waking up in your closet. Here's how to handle them like a pro:

- **Read the label and check the serving size**. Just because the whole bottle looks like a single serving doesn't mean it is. Many drinks are designed to be sipped, not chugged like you're in a college drinking contest.
- **Start low and go slow**. If you don't feel anything right away, don't assume it's not working and take another dose. That's how people end up staring at their hands for three hours wondering if time has stopped. THC drinks take longer to hit than smoking, so patience is key.
- **Don't mix THC drinks with alcohol**. Sure, your THC-infused drink looks like a craft cocktail, but mixing it with alcohol is a terrible idea unless you enjoy unpredictable rollercoasters of intoxication. Crossfading (mixing weed and booze) tends to amplify the effects of both substances, and not in a fun way. Unless you like the feeling of the room spinning, keep your THC drink separate from your whiskey.
- **Stay hydrated and have snacks ready**. THC drinks can cause dry mouth and, don't ignore it, you're going to get hungry. Be prepared. You don't want to be halfway through an existential crisis only to realize you have nothing to eat except that questionable yogurt in the back of your fridge.

Have Fun, But Don't Be an Idiot.

THC drinks are a great alternative to smoking, but they require a little bit of knowledge and self-control. Avoid drinking one right before a work meeting unless you want to find out what your boss really thinks of you when you start grinning for no reason.

Dosing Guide

- 2.5 mg - Mild relaxation, beginner-friendly.
- 5 mg - Noticeable buzz, functional high.
- 10 mg - Stronger effects, best for experienced users.
- 20 mg+ - Buckle up—things are about to get interesting.

Read the label, pace yourself, and don't let impatience turn your fun night into an unplanned journey through the multiverse. Resist the urge to double down just because you don't feel it right away. That's exactly how you end up calling your friend at 2 AM convinced you're stuck in a time loop. Cheers!

> *Pro Tip*: *Make Sure You're in a Good Spot. THC drinks can be fun, relaxing, or unexpectedly intense, so plan accordingly.*

Tinctures & Oils:
The Under-the-Tongue, Grandma-Friendly Option

Tinctures are liquid cannabis extracts that you drop under your tongue for a fast-acting, smoke-free experience. They kick in faster than edibles but don't involve smoking or vaping, making them ideal for people who want precise dosing without committing to the full edible experience.

These are great for:

- People who want precise dosing.
- Medical users.
- Anyone who doesn't want to smell like a reggae festival.

How to Use:

- Drop the oil under your tongue.
- Hold it there for 30-60 seconds (this part is awkward).
- Swallow and wait 15-30 minutes for effects.

✅ Pros of Tinctures & Oils:

- Fast-acting (ish) - Takes effect within 15-30 minutes, much faster than edibles.
- Discreet - No smoke, no smell, just a tiny bottle that looks like medicine. No one knows you're high unless you start giggling uncontrollably.
- Easy to control dosage - You can take as little or as much as you need, no guessing involved. Good for beginners.
- No lung damage - Your doctor will approve.

✖ Cons of Tinctures & Oils:

- Taste can be weird - Some are flavored, but others taste like licking a plant. Not as fun as eating a brownie - Let's be real, tinctures feel like you're taking medicine, not indulging.
- Can be expensive - Quality tinctures aren't cheap, but at least they're reliable.
- Accidentally taking too much, You are in for a surprise edible trip.

If you like precision and don't want to play "Guess the Dosage" with edibles, tinctures are a solid choice.

Topicals: Weed You Can Rub on Your Skin (That Won't Get You High, Sorry)

Topicals are lotions, balms, and creams infused with cannabis that you rub on your skin. They won't get you high (sorry), but they can be great for:

- Muscle pain.
- Inflammation.
- Arthritis.
- Trying to convince your grandma that weed is medicine.

✅ Pros of Topicals:

- No high - Great for people who want relief without tripping out. No high, no paranoia—just pain relief.
- Targeted relief - Perfect for joint pain, arthritis, or that weird knot in your shoulder. Great for medical use.
- Available everywhere - Since they don't contain psychoactive THC (usually), they're legal in more places.
- Non-smelly - Nobody will side-eye you at Thanksgiving.

✗ Cons of Topicals:

- Limited effects - Won't help with anxiety or insomnia, just localized pain.
- Some are overpriced goop - Be wary of fancy CBD creams that cost $100 and do nothing.
- You won't feel a buzz. If you're looking to get high, try literally anything else.

If you're looking for pain relief without the mind-altering fun, topicals are a good option. Just don't expect them to solve all your problems.

Taking Your Ride:
Choose Your Adventure Wisely

Cannabis is fun, helpful, and occasionally life-changing, but it's also wildly unpredictable if you don't know what you're doing. So, there you have it—your cannabis delivery method menu. Whether you want to smoke like a classic stoner, vape like a modern tech bro, risk it all with an edible, or keep it classy with a tincture, there's an option for you.

Pick your method wisely, and for the love of all that is holy, do not be the person who eats an entire edible just because it "didn't kick in yet." The key is to start slow, pay attention, and don't be a hero. Cannabis is fun, useful, and full of possibilities—but only if you use it wisely. Now go forth and experiment (responsibly) and remember: if you find yourself staring at the fridge for 20 minutes trying to remember why you opened it, congratulations—you did it right.

- Start low and slow with edibles and drinks. (Unless you want to meet God.)
- Smoking and vaping are instant but can hit hard.
- Tinctures are subtle but effective.
- Topicals are great for pain, but you won't get high.

Now that you know what it is, how to use it, where to buy legally and how to avoid getting ripped off, it's time to talk about the people you'll meet in the world of cannabis. Spoiler alert: it's not just college kids and tie-dye-wearing hippies. The cannabis culture is packed with characters—from the self-proclaimed strain expert who treats every bud like a fine wine to the old-school stoner still bragging about the "good stuff" from the '70s (even though today's strains would probably launch them into another dimension). Whether you're here for the vibes, the wellness, or just a good time, you're stepping into a community with its own rituals, slang, and unspoken rules. So, let's dive in—welcome to the world of cannabis culture.

Chapter 5: Cannabis Culture – The Good, The Bad, and the Cringeworthy

So, you've familiarized yourself with all the ways to legally (hopefully) acquire and consume cannabis. You've mastered the art of microdosing, figured out that yes, you do have a limit, and hopefully avoided calling 911 because you thought you were dying (spoiler: you weren't).

But cannabis isn't just a product—it's a lifestyle, a community, and for some, a full-blown personality trait. Welcome to the world of cannabis culture, where you'll find everything from highly educated medical users to people who own 47 tie-dye shirts and still think "420 blaze it" is the height of comedy.

This chapter will guide you through the social etiquette, the unspoken rules, and the absolute nonsense you'll have to put up with when you enter the cannabis scene.

The Stereotypes:
Who You'll Meet in the Weed World

Like any subculture, cannabis comes with characters—some delightful, some insufferable. Here's who you're likely to encounter:

The Connoisseur (The Weed Snob).

- Will correct you if you call sativa and indica "strains" instead of "cultivars."
- Owns an actual terpene wheel to analyze the "flavor profile" of their weed.
- Refuses to smoke anything under 25% THC and will look at your pre-roll like it's a gas station hot dog.
- Can tell you the exact farm, soil composition, and farmer's astrological sign for their preferred bud.

Usefulness: High (pun intended). They know their stuff, but beware—you may never enjoy "regular" weed again after talking to them.

The "It's Just a Plant, Man" Guy.

- Believes weed can cure everything, including cancer, heartbreak, and bad credit scores.
- Thinks "Big Pharma" is suppressing *the truth* about cannabis (not entirely wrong, but calm down).
- Refers to cannabis as a "sacred medicine" but has absolutely zero medical knowledge.
- Has a Bob Marley poster. (It's required.)

Usefulness: Medium. Good for vibes, terrible for science.

The Dispensary Bro.

- Works at a dispensary and acts like he's curing disease and solving world hunger.
- Talks way too much about "terps" and "entourage effects."
- Calls himself a budtender like he's an actual pharmacist.
- Will absolutely sell you something too strong for your tolerance level.

Usefulness: Dangerous. Proceed with caution.

The Paranoid First-Timer *(You, Probably)*.

- Asks, "Am I too high?" every two minutes.
- Thinks the cops are coming (even though it's legal).
- Checks their pulse at least four times.
- Texts a friend: "How long does this last???" (Answer: Longer than you'd like.)

Usefulness: None. You're useless right now. Just ride it out.

Weed Etiquette:
Don't Be "That Person"

Now that you've met the cast of characters, it's time to discuss how to behave when partaking in cannabis. Yes, even weed has rules.

The Golden Rules of Sharing Weed.

- Puff, Puff, Pass. Don't hog the joint unless you enjoy being side-eyed into oblivion.
- Don't "Wet-Lip" the Joint. This isn't a makeout session—keep it dry.
- Corner the Bowl. If using a pipe, don't torch the entire thing. Be considerate and light just the edge.

- Don't Be a Weed Mooch. If you never bring your own, people *will* notice.
- Respect the Host's Rules. If they say, "no smoking inside," don't be *that guy* lighting up next to their scented candles.

How to Avoid a Weed-Induced Existential Crisis.

- Know Your Limit. The goal is to relax, not to have a full-blown meltdown about the meaning of life.
- Don't Mix with Alcohol Until You Know What You're Doing. Unless you like feeling like you're on a carnival ride that won't stop.
- If You Get Too High, DO NOT Call 911. Just drink some water, watch cartoons, and accept your fate.

> *Warning*: *If you're hitting a joint, do not slobber all over it. This is a smoke session, not a kissing booth.*

Buying Weed
Without Looking Like a Total Newb

Dispensaries are not the Wild West anymore—they're sleek, corporate, and shockingly expensive. Here's how to blend in and not look like it's your first time.

- Know What You Want. Don't stand at the counter looking confused while people behind you sigh dramatically.
- Ask for Recommendations (Without Sounding Clueless). Instead of "What's good?" try, "I'm looking for something mellow but uplifting, any recommendations?"
- Avoid the Cheapest Weed. There's a reason that $15 eighth smells like wet hay and disappointment.

- Don't Get Pressured into Buying More. Dispensary staff love upselling. You do not need a 100mg edible unless you're trying to astral project.

> *Pro Tip*: *Walking into a dispensary and saying, "Uh, I just want weed" is like going to a bar and saying, "I just want alcohol." Be specific unless you want the budtender to sigh at you dramatically.*

The Legal Side:
"Wait, Can I Actually Do This?"

This is where things get tricky. Just because cannabis is legal in some places doesn't mean you can do whatever you want. Here are some ways you can still get into trouble:

- **Crossing State Lines**: Just because it's legal in California doesn't mean you can take it to Texas. The TSA does not care about your weed gummies.
- **Driving While High**: It's still a DUI, even if you were just "a little relaxed."
- **Public Consumption**: Smoking a joint in a park might seem chill, but legally, it's the same as drinking in public— illegal in most places.
- **Mailing Weed**: The feds still consider cannabis illegal, so if you think sending your grandma an edible care package is cute—don't.
- **Your Employer Can Still Fire You**: Just because it's legal doesn't mean your boss won't say, "Yeah, no."

You're Not Alone:
Welcome to the Weed Community

You're officially one of us now. That's right—welcome to the club. Cannabis culture is weird, wonderful, and occasionally insufferable. You will meet people who treat it like fine wine and others who act like it's a personality replacement. Weed people are everywhere: your barista, your accountant, your grandma (don't ask questions). Whether you're in it for wellness or just here for the giggles, you're part of a global community that loves this plant—and argues endlessly about it.

There are online groups like "High Society: Cannabis Users" where stoners, skeptics, and curious rookies swap advice, debate terpenes, and share memes about edibles hitting too hard. Some folks treat cannabis like fine wine; others just want to stop overthinking at bedtime. There's room for both.

Just be warned: now that you're in, you'll have to survive the eternal sativa vs. indica debate, cringe at the corporate sellouts in cannabis, and pretend not to care whether Willie Nelson is actually immortal. (He is. Obviously.)

You've made it this far—congratulations! By now, you should have a solid grasp on the essentials: how to buy legally without ending up in handcuffs, how to find the right dispensary without getting scammed, and how to navigate the cannabis culture without looking completely clueless. But before you embark on your green journey, we've got a few final tips to make sure you actually enjoy the ride.

So, let's wrap it all up, throw in some last-minute wisdom, and send you off with the confidence of a seasoned pro (or at least someone who won't embarrass themselves on their first trip to the dispensary).

Important: Weed culture is welcoming, but public smoking is still illegal in most places. Yes, even you think it "totally smells like a skunk."

Conclusion: So, Now You're a Weed Expert (Sort Of)

Congratulations! You've made it through this book without accidentally hotboxing your grandma's bathroom or calling the cops on yourself after eating a 10mg gummy. That alone deserves a round of applause. You are now (at least on paper) an informed, responsible, and totally *chill* cannabis consumer. Or, at the very least, you've absorbed enough information to avoid looking like an absolute fool at the dispensary.

But before you run off into the sunset with your newly acquired vape pen and a smug sense of enlightenment, let's take a moment to reflect on what you've learned.

You're Probably Still Going to Mess Up at Some Point

At this point, you've learned the basics. You're prepped, you're ready, and hopefully, you're not about to pull a 'first-time disaster special.' But let's go over the golden rule one last time: never get high alone your first time. It's like going skydiving without an instructor or watching a horror movie alone in a cabin—technically doable, but do you really want to take that risk? Stick with your trusted people, don't wander off into the night like an unchaperoned toddler, and for the love of all things holy, never let go of your wingman.

Let's be real. No matter how many times I've told you to respect the edibles, there's a *very* high chance (pun intended) that you'll still end up sitting on your couch, clutching a bag of Doritos, contemplating your entire life's decisions because that 5mg gummy "wasn't working" so you took three more.

And you know what? That's fine. Everyone needs that *one* experience where they stare at the ceiling for four hours wondering if they can hear colors. Consider it a rite of passage.

> *Warning*: If you ignore everything else, at least remember this—do not take a 100mg edible just because "it's not working yet." You will regret it.

Weed Won't Fix Everything
(But It Might Help You Tolerate It Better)

Look, cannabis is great, but let's not pretend it's a magical cure-all. Will it make your anxiety disappear? *Maybe.* Will it turn you into a productivity machine? *Doubtful.* Will it make family holidays slightly more tolerable? *Absolutely.*

The key is balance—a concept that, let's be honest, most people who just discovered weed have *zero* grasp of. But hey, at least now you *know* that smoking a whole joint before a work meeting is probably not the best idea (unless you work at a drum circle).

You Will Now Start Judging Others
(and That's Okay)

Once you've dipped your toes into the world of cannabis, it's only natural to start developing strong opinions. You'll spot the *amateur move* from a mile away:

- The person who takes an edible before a long-haul flight and forgets they're trapped in a flying tube of existential horror.
- The overconfident newbie who claims they have a "super high tolerance" and then proceeds to melt into the couch like a forgotten ice cream cone.
- The guy at the party who won't stop talking about the entourage effect even though nobody asked.

You'll see them. You'll recognize them. And you'll smile, knowing that you were *once* one of them.

The Legal System Is Still a Mess, So Be Careful

If you take *nothing else* from this book, let it be this: Just because it's legal somewhere doesn't mean you can be reckless.

- Transporting weed across state lines? Still illegal.
- Getting high and then trying to explain to a cop that "it's just a plant, man"? Bad idea.
- Assuming your employer is "totally chill" because your boss has a beard and wears Birkenstocks? Rookie mistake.

Seriously, stay informed, stay cautious, and for the love of everything holy, do not get arrested because you thought a CBD vape was a "legal loophole."

You're Officially One of Us Now
(Welcome to the Club)

The good news? You've joined a massive, ever-growing community of cannabis users—some responsible, some... well, not so much. You'll soon discover that weed people are *everywhere*—your coworkers, your barista, your elderly neighbor who *definitely* bakes her own edibles.

You can now join our Facebook Group "High society: Cannabis Users" at **www.facebook.com/groups/highsocietyweed/**. The world of cannabis can be confusing, but we make it simple! Whether you're exploring THC & CBD for wellness, looking for dispensary tips, or just want real talk about what works with fellow minded Cannabis curious people—this is your safe space.

The bad news? You'll now have to endure the endless, insufferable debates about indica vs. sativa, the ethics of big cannabis corporations, and whether or not Willie Nelson is actually immortal.

Then again, that's part of the fun. So go forth, smoke responsibly, and remember: if you ever find yourself too high, just drink some water, take a nap, and accept your terrible decisions. You'll be fine. Probably.

Important: Just because you finished this book does not mean you're ready to out-smoke Snoop Dogg. Stay in your lane, rookie.

Your Final Tip:
Don't Forget to Tip Your Budtender

Seriously—tip your budtender, they put up with *so much nonsense*. They deal with confused tourists, overconfident stoners, and people who still think "kush" is a new kind of energy drink. If they help you pick the right edible or save you from accidentally buying concentrate when you meant to get a vape cartridge, that's worth a couple bucks.

Treat them like the cannabis spirit guides they are, and your next visit might just come with better service and zero judgment when you forget what you came in for.

The key to enjoying cannabis? Find what works for you, don't be a mooch, and for the love of all things holy, RESPECT THE EDIBLES.

Now go forth, be responsible, and please—don't be the person who eats an entire edible because they "didn't feel anything yet." The world has enough of those already.

Appendix
State Chart as of June 2025.

As of June 2025, the legal status of cannabis in the United States varies by state, encompassing aspects such as medical use, recreational use, possession limits, cultivation rights, and product-specific regulations. Below is a basic overview of each state's stance on cannabis:

We break this down into 5 categories for each state:

- Recreation: Is Recreational use legal?
- Medical: Is Medical use legal?
- Carry: How much can you possess or have on you?
- (Medical): How much can you have for medical purposes?
- Home Grown: Are you able to grow your own?
- Notes: Under each state we have listed basic notes on the status of the law in that state.

REMEMBER: laws are always changing, and this is a basic table. We are not your attorney or legal expert so check with your state before relying on information here that may be old or outdated. For the most recent chart go to www.RonanBlaschko.com to download. (Although considering this is a book about marijuana, we'll update it as soon as we get to it, wink, wink).

State	Recreation	Medical	Carry	(Medical)	Home Grown

Notes

Alabama	Illegal	Legal	N/A	"70/day	Illegal

Medical use legalized in May 2021; first-time possession may be a misdemeanor; subsequent offenses are felonies. "70/day dosages" refers to the maximum amount a patient can possess at one time.

Alaska	Legal	Legal	1oz	1oz	Yes

Recreational use legalized by Measure 2 in 2014; Cultivate six plants, with no more than three mature at a time.

Arizona	Legal	Legal	1oz	2.5oz/14 days	Yes

Recreational use legalized in 2020; Cultivate six plants, with a maximum of twelve plants/household.

Arkansas	Illegal	Legal	N/A	2.5oz/14 days	No

Medical use legalized in 2016; recreational use remains illegal.

California	Legal	Legal	1oz	8oz	Yes

Recreational use legalized by Proposition 64 in 2016; Cultivate six plants/residence.

Colorado	Legal	Legal	1oz	2oz	Yes

Recreational use legalized by Amendment 64 in 2012; Cultivate six plants, with no more than three mature at a time.

Connecticut	Legal	Legal	1.5oz	3oz	Yes

Recreational use legalized in 2021; Cultivate six plants, with a maximum of twelve/household.

Delaware	Legal	Legal	1oz	6oz	No

Recreational use legalized in 2023; HB☐110 (April 2025) stricter FBI background for cannabis business licenses. Home cultivation is not permitted.

Florida	Illegal	Legal	N/A	2.5oz/35 days	No

Medical use legalized 2016; recreational failed 11/24. Ballot initiative in 2026.

Georgia	Illegal	Limited	N/A	Low-THC oil (20oz)	No

Only low-THC oil (less than 5% THC) is permitted for specific medical conditions.

Hawaii	Decrim	Legal	3g(Decrim)	4oz	Yes

Possession of 3 grams is Decrim; medical use legalized in 2000; patients can cultivate ten plants. Recreational Bill May Pass in 2025/2026.

State	Recreation	Medical	Carry	(Medical)	Home Grown

Notes

Idaho	Illegal	Illegal	N/A	N/A	No

Both medical and recreational use are illegal, but activists have begun signature collection for medical use in 2026.

Illinois	Legal	Legal	30 g	2.5oz	No

Recreational use legalized in 2019; home cultivation is permitted only for medical patients (five plants).

Indiana	Illegal	Illegal	N/A	N/A	No

Both medical and recreational use are illegal.

Iowa	Illegal	Limited	N/A	4.5g THC/90 days	No

Only low-THC medical cannabis is permitted for specific conditions.

Kansas	Illegal	Illegal	N/A	N/A	No

Both medical and recreational use are illegal.

Kentucky	Illegal	Legal	N/A	30-day supply	No

Full medical program began Jan 2025; smokable forms still banned.

Louisiana	Illegal	Legal	N/A	2.5oz/14 days	No

Medical use legalized in 2015; recreational use remains illegal.

Maine	Legal	Legal	2.5oz	2.5oz	Yes

Recreational use legalized in 2016; Cultivate three mature plants.

Maryland	Legal	Legal	1.5oz	120 g	Yes

Recreational use legalized in 2022; Cultivate two plants/person, with a maximum of four/residence.

Massachusetts	Legal	Legal	1oz-10oz home	10oz	Yes

Recreational use legalized in 2016; Cultivate six plants, with a maximum of twelve/household.

Michigan	Legal	Legal	2.5oz/10 home	2.5oz	Yes

Recreational use legalized in 2018; Cultivate twelve plants/household.

Minnesota	Legal	Legal	2oz (8g conc.)	2.5oz	Yes

Recreational use legalized in 2023; Cultivate eight plants, with 4 mature max. 2025 bill clarifies medical reciprocity and labeling; no major changes.

State	Recreation	Medical	Carry	(Medical)	Home Grown
Mississippi	Illegal	Legal	N/A	3.5 g/day	No

Medical use legalized in 2022; recreational use remains illegal.

| Missouri | Legal | Legal | 3oz | 4oz/30 days | Yes |

Recreational use legalized in 2022; Cultivate six flowering plants with a cultivation card.

| Montana | Legal | Legal | 1oz | 1oz | Yes |

Recreational use legalized in 2020; Cultivate 4/person, 8 max/household. SB 27 freezes new license apps after June 30, 2025.

| Nebraska | Illegal | Illegal | N/A | N/A | No |

Both medical and recreational use are illegal; possession of small amounts is Decrim, resulting in a civil infraction. Medical legalization efforts for 2026 ballot.

| Nevada | Legal | Legal | 1oz (3.5g conc.) | 2.5oz | Yes |

Recreational use legalized in 2016; Cultivate six plants/person, with a maximum of twelve/household, only if there is no retail cannabis store within 25 miles of the home.

| New Hampshire | Decrim | Legal | 3/4oz (Decrim) | 2oz | No |

Possession of 3/4 ounce is Decriminalized; medical use legalized in 2013; recreational use remains illegal, but limited legalization bill under review.

| New Jersey | Legal | Legal | 6oz | 3oz/30 days | No |

Recreational use legalized in 2020; home cultivation is not permitted.

| New Mexico | Legal | Legal | 2oz | 8oz/90 days | Yes |

Recreational use legalized in 2021; Cultivate six mature plants, with a maximum of twelve/household.

| New York | Legal | Legal | 3oz-24g conc | 60-day supply | Yes |

Recreational use legalized in 2021; Cultivate six plants/person, with a maximum of twelve/household.

| North Carolina | Illegal | Illegal | N/A | N/A | No |

Both medical and recreational use are illegal; possession of small amounts is Decriminalized, resulting in a civil infraction.

State	Recreation	Medical	Carry	(Medical)	Home Grown

Notes

State	Recreation	Medical	Carry	(Medical)	Home Grown
North Dakota	Illegal	Legal	N/A	3oz	No

Medical use legalized in 2016; recreational use remains illegal.

Ohio	Legal	Legal	2.5oz	90-day supply	Yes

Recreational use legal since Dec 2023; Cultivate 6 plants.

Oklahoma	Illegal	Legal	N/A	3oz	Yes

Medical use legalized in 2018; recreational use remains illegal; patients can cultivate six mature plants.

Oregon	Legal	Legal	2oz/1 public	24oz	Yes

Recreational use legalized in 2014; Cultivate four plants/residence.

Pennsylvania	Illegal	Legal	N/A	30-day supply	No

Medical use legalized in 2016; recreational use remains illegal, but bipartisan medical expansion & rec talks.

Rhode Island	Legal	Legal	1oz	2.5oz	Yes

Recreational use legalized in 2022; Cultivate six plants, with a maximum of three mature at a time.

South Carolina	Illegal	Illegal	N/A	N/A	No

Both medical and recreational use are illegal.

South Dakota	Illegal	Legal	N/A	3oz	No

Medical use legalized in 2021; recreational use remains illegal, but recreational ballot attempt in 2026.

Tennessee	Illegal	Limited	N/A	Low-THC oil	No

Only low-THC oil is permitted for medical use under specific conditions.

Texas	Illegal	Limited	N/A	Low-THC oil	No

SB 3 bans hemp-derived THC starting Sept 2025; low-THC medical use allowed.

Utah	Illegal	Legal	N/A	113 g	No

Medical use legalized in 2018; recreational use remains illegal.

Vermont	Legal	Legal	1oz	2oz	Yes

Recreational use legalized in 2018; Cultivate two mature plants and four immature plants/residence.

State	Recreation	Medical	Carry	(Medical)	Home Grown
Virginia	Legal	Legal	1oz	4oz	Yes

Recreational use legalized in 2021; Cultivate four plants/household. Retail sales licensed Sept 2025; stores open May 2026 per new law.

| Washington | Legal | Legal | 1oz | 3oz | No |

Recreational use legalized in 2012; home cultivation is permitted only for medical patients (six plants).

| West Virginia | Illegal | Legal | N/A | 30-day supply | No |

Medical use legalized in 2017; recreational use remains illegal.

| Wisconsin | Illegal | Illegal | N/A | N/A | No |

Both medical and recreational use are illegal; possession of small amounts may be a misdemeanor. Bill unlikely in 2025, but 2026 elections could flip balance.

| Wyoming | Illegal | Illegal | N/A | N/A | No |

Both medical and recreational use are illegal; possession of small amounts is a misdemeanor.